Global surveillance, prevention and control of CHRONIC RESPIRATORY DISEASES

A comprehensive approach

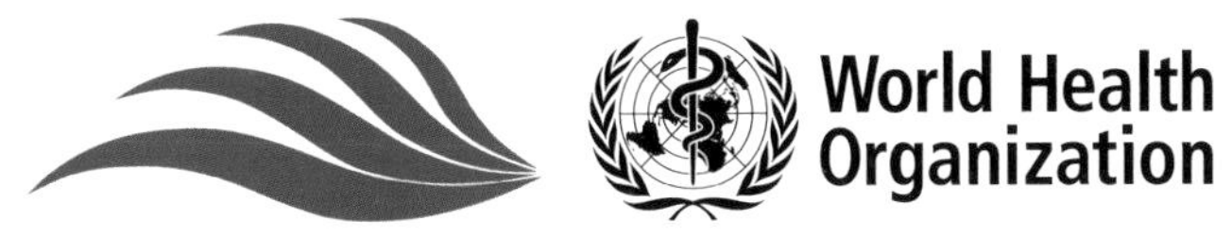

WHO Library Cataloguing-in-Publication Data:

Global surveillance, prevention and control of chronic respiratory diseases : a comprehensive approach / Jean Bousquet and Nikolai Khaltaev editors.

1.Respiratory tract diseases - epidemiology. 2 Respiratory tract diseases - etiology. 3.Pulmonary disease, Chronic obstructive - epidemiology. 4. Pulmonary disease, Chronic obstructive - etiology 5.Risk factors. 6.Chronic disease -prevention and control 7.Strategic planning. 8.Health policy. I.World Health Organization. II.Bousquet, Jean. III.Khaltaev, Nikolai. IV.Title: A world where all people breathe freely.

ISBN 978 92 4 156346 8 (NLM classification: WF 140)

Printed in Switzerland

This publication was produced under the overall direction of Jean Bousquet and Nikolai Khaltaev (Editors).

The core contributors were Alvaro A. Cruz, Eva Mantzouranis (2003-2006), Paolo M. Matricardi (2002-2005) and Elisabetta Minelli (World Health Organization); Nadia Aït-Khaled, Eric D. Bateman, Carlos Baena-Cagnani, Michael Boland, Sonia A. Buist, G. Walter Canonica, Kai-Hakon Carlsen, Ronald Dahl, Leonardo M. Fabbri, Yoshinosuke Fukuchi, Lawrence Grouse, Marc Humbert, Claude Lenfant, Jean Luc Malo, Walter T. McNicholas, Ruby Pawankar, Klaus F. Rabe, F. Estelle R. Simons, Archie Turnbull, Erkka Valovirta, Paul van Cauwenberge, Giovanni Viegi, Chris Van Weel, Sally Wenzel and Nanshan Zhong.

Valuable inputs in the form of contributions, peer-review, suggestions and criticisms were received from Tim Armstrong, Michal Krzyzanowski, Doris Ma Fat, Salah-Eddine Ottmani, Annette Pruess-Ustun, Eva Rehfuess, Luminita Sanda and Kenji Shibuya (World Health Organization); Ali Ben Kheder, Paulo Camargos, Yu Zhi Chen, Alexander Chuchalin, Peter M. Calverley, Adnan Custovic, Habib Douagui, Wytske J. Fokkens, Amiran Gamkrelidze, Tari Haahtela, Suzanne Hurd, Abai Kabatayevich Baigenzhin, You-Young Kim, Ali Kocabas, Carlos Luna, Fernando D. Martinez, Sylvia Mavale-Manuel, Mário Moraes de Almeida, Paul O'Byrne, Solange Ouedraogo, James P. Kiley, Rogelio Perez-Padilla, Todor Popov, Jose Rosado-Pinto, Kazimierz Roszkowski-Pliz, Alkis Togias, Arzu Yorgancioglu, Mahamad Yousser and Osman Yusuf.

Editorial revision was done by Angela Haden and Pieter Desloovere.

Book: design and layout, Zando F. Escultura; cover: design and layout, Reda Sadki; pictures: Marko Kokic (cover), Patrick Szymshek (Pelé) and George Herringshaw (Rosa Mota).

Report development and production were coordinated by Pieter Desloovere who also was responsible for the web site version.

The Global Alliance against Chronic Respiratory Diseases wishes to thank the following for their generous financial support: GlaxoSmithKline, Nycomed-Altana Pharma US, Inc., Chiesi Farmaceutici S.p.A, Merck & Co. Inc, Pfizer Inc., Schering Plough Corporation, Astra Zeneca R&D Lund, Boehringer-Ingelheim Int. GmbH, Novartis Pharma AG, Sanofi-Aventis and Stallergènes SA.

CONTENTS

FOREWORD

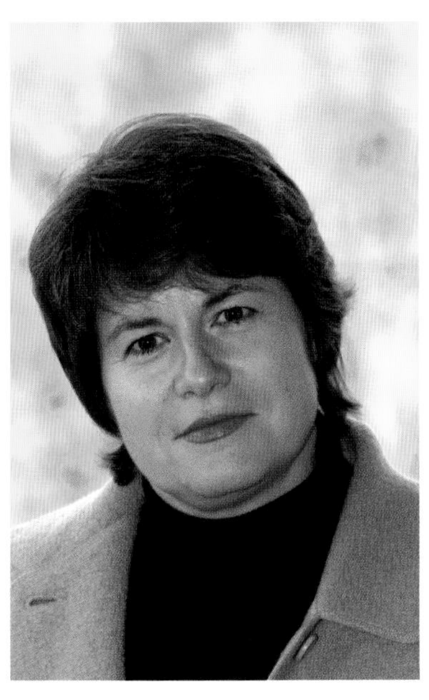

Chronic respiratory diseases, such as asthma and chronic obstructive pulmonary disease, kill more than four million people every year and affect hundreds of millions more. These diseases erode the health and well-being of the patients and have a negative impact on families and societies. Women and children are particularly vulnerable, especially those in low and middle income countries, where they are exposed on a daily basis to indoor air pollution from solid fuels for cooking and heating. In high income countries, tobacco is the most important risk factor for chronic respiratory diseases, and in some of these countries, tobacco use among women and young people is still increasing.

WHO recently launched the Global Alliance against Chronic Respiratory Diseases (GARD). Spearheaded by WHO, GARD brings together the combined knowledge of national and international organizations, institutions and agencies to improve the lives of millions of people affected by chronic respiratory diseases.

Global Surveillance, prevention and control of chronic respiratory diseases: a comprehensive approach raises awareness of the huge impact of chronic respiratory diseases worldwide, and highlights the risk factors as well as ways to prevent and treat these diseases.

I hope that this publication will serve not only as a source of information, but also as inspiration to those who want to join the battle against chronic respiratory diseases. By addressing this global epidemic, much suffering can be avoided and millions of lives can be saved.

Dr Catherine Le Galès-Camus
WHO Assistant Director-General,
Noncommunicable Diseases and Mental Health

SUPPORTING STATEMENTS

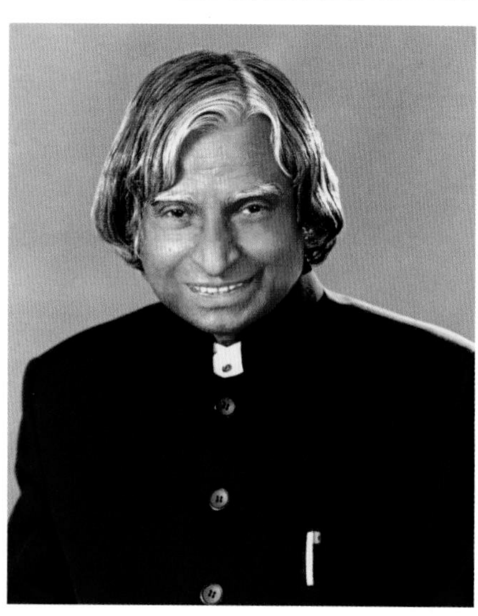

Better surveillance to map the magnitude of chronic respiratory diseases with reference to needy persons and the disadvantaged is required. Chronic respiratory diseases which are preventable, especially affect the elderly and children. *Global surveillance, prevention and control of chronic respiratory diseases: a comprehensive approach* should be a practical guide on the good principles which can be followed by patients and the public at large. I extend my greetings and felicitations to all those associated with this mission and wish the Global Alliance against Chronic Respiratory Diseases all success.

A.P.J. Abdul Kalam
Past-President of the Republic of India

Reaching a major goal like conquering chronic respiratory diseases is similar to a marathon run: it's a big effort but with energy, knowledge, support and the will to win, it can be done. I am convinced that the Global Alliance against Chronic Respiratory Diseases will win the battle against chronic respiratory disease, which kills four million people a year.

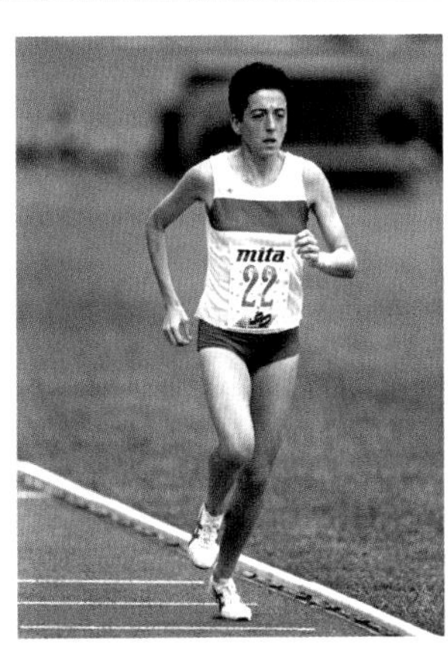

Rosa Mota
Marathon runner and Olympic marathon champion, Portugal

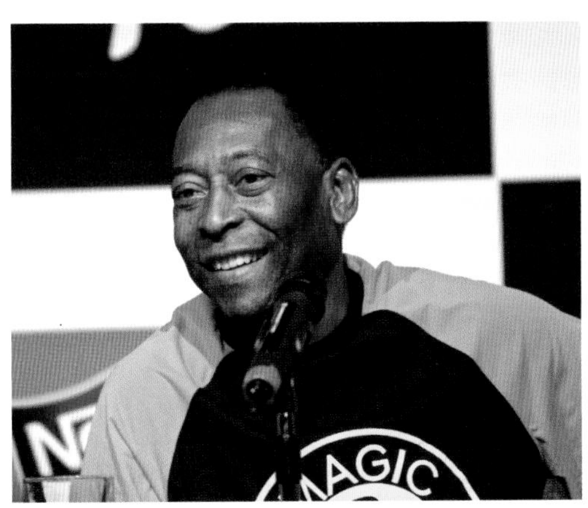

I am happy to hear that the Global Alliance against Chronic Respiratory Diseases is now in place as a global team. As a team, each member will contribute his or her unique strengths, just like in football. Together, the Alliance's teamwork will provide help to the hundreds of millions of people who suffer from chronic respiratory diseases, including those in my country who do not have access to essential treatments.

Edson Arantes do Nascimento, Pelé
Football legend, Brazil

OVERVIEW

1. The Burden of Chronic Diseases

KEY MESSAGES

- **80% of chronic disease deaths occur in low and middle income countries.**
- **The threat is growing – the number of people, families and communities afflicted is increasing.**
- **This growing threat is an under-appreciated cause of poverty and retards the economic development of many countries.**
- **The chronic disease threat can be overcome using existing knowledge.**
- **The solutions are effective – and highly cost effective.**
- **Comprehensive and integrated action at country level, led by governments, is the means to achieve success.**

Chronic diseases are the major cause of premature adult deaths in all regions of the world. Yet they have generally been neglected on the international health and development agenda. The global report on chronic diseases from the World Health Organization (WHO) presents current data on the burden of disease, and makes the case for increased and urgent action to prevent and control chronic diseases (*1, 2*).

In his foreword to the report (*1*), Dr LEE Jong-Wook, the late Director-General of WHO, declared: "The lives of too many people in the world are being blighted and cut short by chronic diseases such as heart disease, stroke, cancer, chronic respiratory diseases and diabetes." There is an urgent need to prevent and control chronic diseases within the context of international health.

Chronic diseases were estimated to account for 35 million (*2*), of a projected total of 58 million deaths from all causes in 2005. Chronic diseases account for twice as many deaths as all communicable diseases (including HIV/AIDS, tuberculosis and malaria), maternal and perinatal conditions, and nutritional deficiencies combined (Figure 1). Only 20% of cases of chronic disease occur in high income countries.

For the next 10–20 years, communicable diseases will remain the predominant health problem for the populations in low income countries. However, an epidemic of chronic diseases is expected to occur in the future in all countries, including low and middle income countries (*3–5*).

Collecting information on non-fatal health outcomes of disease and injury has often been neglected in health planning because of the conceptual complexity of measuring morbidity and disability in populations, and the difficulty of defining terms. To overcome these difficulties, disability-adjusted life years (DALYs), which combine morbidity and mortality (see Box 1), were launched by the World Bank and backed by WHO as a measure of the global burden of disease (*6*).

Box 1 Disability-adjusted life years (DALYs)

- **One DALY represents the loss of the equivalent of one year of full health.**
- **DALYs for a disease are the sum of the years of life lost as a result of premature mortality in the population and the years lost as a result of disability for incident cases of the health condition.**
- **The DALY is a health gap measure that extends the concept of potential years of life lost as a result of premature death to include equivalent years of "healthy" life lost in states of less than full health, broadly termed disability.**

Source: reference *7*.

Although the DALY method may be subject to some criticism (*8*), it allows for comprehensive, consistent and comparable information on diseases and injuries. DALYs may be used as a health indicator allowing for surveillance and evaluation of overall health. Chronic diseases represent an important part of DALYs worldwide (Figure 1).

Figure 1 Projected global deaths and disability–adjusted life years (DALYs) in 2005

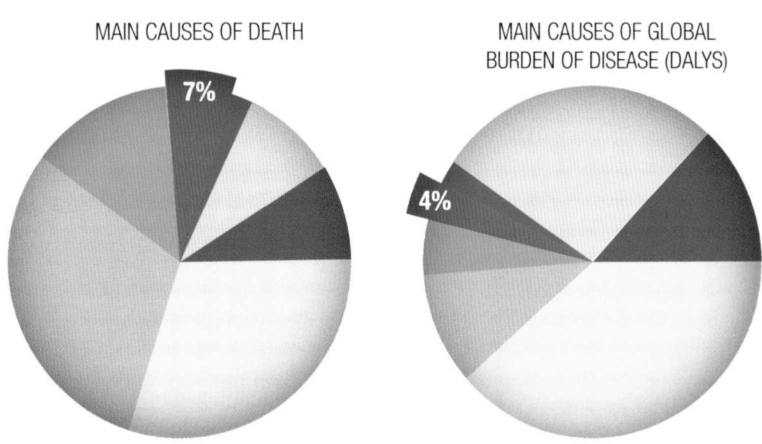

- Communicable diseases, maternal and perinatal conditions, nutritional deficiencies
- Cardiovascular disease
- Cancer
- Chronic respiratory diseases
- Diabetes
- Other chronic diseases
- Injuries

Source: reference *1*.

Figure 2 Projected main causes of disability–adjusted life years (DALYs), by income (all ages, 2005)

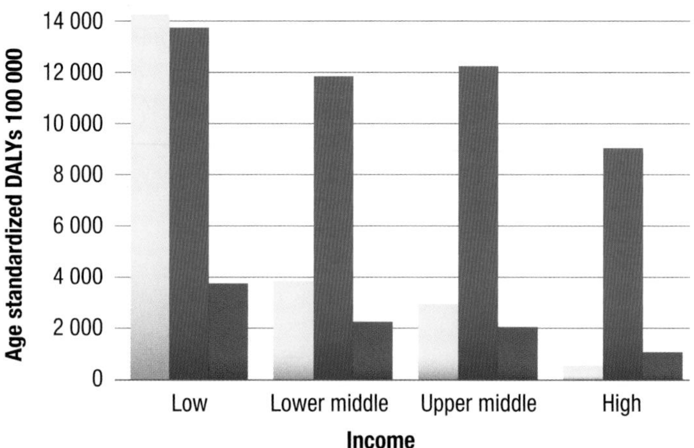

Communicable diseases, maternal and perinatal conditions, nutritional deficiencies
Chronic diseases
Injuries

Source: reference *1*.

Assuming that no pandemic occurs, deaths from infectious diseases, maternal and perinatal conditions, and nutritional deficiencies combined are projected to decline by 3% over the next 10 years. In the same period, deaths attributable to chronic diseases are projected to increase by 17%.

Chronic diseases hinder economic growth and reduce the development potential of countries, in particular the poorest ones. However, chronic diseases have generally been neglected in international health and development work (*9*). They were not included among the global Millennium Development Goal (MDG) targets.

Chronic diseases and poverty

Chronic diseases and poverty are interconnected in a vicious cycle (*10*). The reasons for this are clear (Figure 3).

In almost all countries, the poorest people are the most at risk for developing chronic respiratory diseases. The poorest people are also most likely to die prematurely from these diseases because of greater exposure to risks and decreased access to health services. For example, in children with asthma, poverty aggravates asthma and asthma aggravates poverty. People with

Figure 3 From poverty to chronic disease

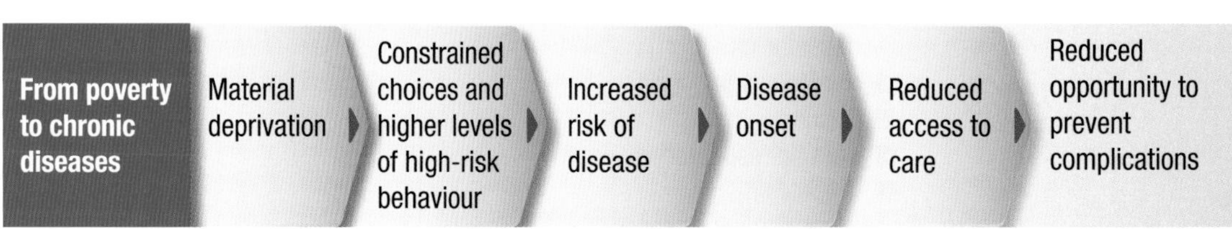
From poverty to chronic diseases
Material deprivation
Constrained choices and higher levels of high-risk behaviour
Increased risk of disease
Disease onset
Reduced access to care
Reduced opportunity to prevent complications

Source: reference *1*.

asthma are less able to work or look after their families. Children with asthma are likely to miss a significant part of their education. Drug costs, emergency visits, hospitalization and inappropriate treatments are a huge financial drain on struggling health systems.

For various reasons, tobacco use tends to be higher among poor people than among wealthier members of society, and poorer people therefore spend relatively more on tobacco products. In low and middle income countries, poor people are more exposed to indoor solid fuels and to unsafe occupational environments.

Chronic diseases also have an indirect impact on people's economic status and employment opportunities in the long term (*1, 11*). Indirect costs include:

- Reduction in income owing to loss of productivity as a result of illness or death.
- The earnings of adult household members forgone by caring for those who are ill.
- Reduction in future earnings by the selling of assets to cope with direct costs and unpredictable expenditures.
- Lost opportunities for young members of the household who leave school in order to care for adults who are ill or who go to work to help the household economy.

These costs are significant in high income countries where people are protected by social security systems. Even in these countries, not all patients can afford expensive medical services. However, these costs are devastating in low and middle income countries where insurance systems are either underdeveloped or nonexistent. For example, in Burkina Faso chronic diseases represent one of the major causes of catastrophic expenditure (any health expenditure that threatens a household's financial capacity to meet its subsistence needs) (*12*).

Chronic respiratory diseases in particular place a grave economic burden on countries because of the major effect of occupational lung diseases. This burden will increase if no action is taken. The evidence is clear. Action is urgently needed to avoid an adverse impact on national economic development.

2. Preventable Chronic Respiratory Diseases: A Major Global Health Problem

KEY MESSAGES

- **Chronic respiratory diseases are chronic diseases of the airways and the other structures of the lungs. Major preventable chronic respiratory diseases include asthma and respiratory allergies, chronic obstructive pulmonary disease (COPD), occupational lung diseases, sleep apnea syndrome and pulmonary hypertension.**
- **Hundreds of millions of people of all ages (from infancy to old age) suffer from preventable chronic respiratory diseases and respiratory allergies in all countries of the world.**
- **More than 500 million of these people live in low and middle income countries or deprived populations.**
- **Chronic respiratory diseases account for four million deaths annually.**
- **Measured in DALYs, in 2005 the burden of chronic respiratory diseases was projected to account for 4% of the global burden and 8.3% of the burden of chronic diseases.**
- **Preventable chronic respiratory diseases are increasing in prevalence, particularly among children and elderly people.**
- **The burden of preventable chronic respiratory diseases has major adverse effects on the quality of life and disability of affected individuals.**
- **Many risk factors for preventable chronic respiratory diseases have been identified and efficient preventive measures established.**
- **Effective management plans have been shown to reduce the morbidity and mortality caused by chronic respiratory diseases.**
- **Prevention and management plans concerning chronic respiratory diseases are fragmented and need to be coordinated.**

The health of the world is generally improving. Fewer people are dying from infectious diseases and therefore in many cases are living long enough to develop chronic diseases (*1*).

Chronic respiratory diseases, chronic diseases of the airways and the other structures of the lungs, represent a wide array of serious diseases. Preventable chronic respiratory diseases include asthma and respiratory allergies, chronic obstructive pulmonary disease (COPD), occupational lung diseases, sleep apnea syndrome and pulmonary hypertension. They constitute a serious public health problem in all countries throughout the world, in particular in low and middle income countries and in deprived populations.

Hundreds of millions of people of all ages, in all countries of the world, are affected by preventable chronic respiratory diseases. More than 50% of them live in low and middle income countries or deprived populations. The prevalence of preventable chronic respiratory diseases is increasing everywhere and in particular among children and elderly people.

The burden of preventable chronic respiratory diseases has major adverse effects on the quality of life and disability of affected individuals. Preventable chronic respiratory diseases cause premature deaths. They also have large adverse and underappreciated economic effects on families, communities and societies in general.

Many risk factors for preventable chronic respiratory diseases have been identified:

- Tobacco smoke and other forms of indoor air pollution, particularly in low and middle income countries.
- Allergens.
- Occupational agents.
- Diseases such as schistosomiasis or sickle cell disease.
- Living at a high altitude.

Prevention of these risk factors will have a significant impact on morbidity and mortality. Efficient preventive measures exist. Yet, preventable chronic respiratory diseases and their risk factors receive insufficient attention from the health-care community, government officials, patients and their families as well as the media (Table 1). Preventable chronic respiratory diseases are under-recognized, under-diagnosed, under-treated and insufficiently prevented.

Barriers increasing the burden of chronic respiratory diseases

Several barriers have been shown to reduce the availability, affordability, dissemination and efficacy of optimal management of chronic respiratory diseases (*13–15*):

- Economic and generic barriers include poverty, poor education, illiteracy, lack of sanitation and poor infrastructure.
- Cultural barriers include multiplicity of languages, as well as religious and cultural beliefs.

Table 1 Barriers that increase the burden of chronic respiratory diseases

	Low and middle income countries	High income countries
Insufficient priority	In many low and middle income countries, the focus of health-care systems is on communicable diseases and injuries. Infrastructure for the diagnosis and management of chronic respiratory diseases is either not available or is viewed as low priority on any public health agenda.	Chronic respiratory diseases are usually independent of communicable diseases in terms of public health management, and there are structures for fighting both types of diseases. A few successful national programmes against chronic respiratory diseases exist. However, they are not comprehensive (e.g. there are programmes dealing with asthma or COPD), they are fragmented, need to be expanded and integrated within a single action plan and they require more coordination. Moreover, chronic respiratory diseases are rarely on the public health agenda.
	Data on chronic respiratory disease risk factors, burden and surveillance are scarce or unavailable in most countries. Consequently the true burden of chronic respiratory diseases on health services and society is not appreciated.	Data on the chronic respiratory disease risk factors, burden and surveillance are fragmented and often incomplete.
	Strategies for the prevention of chronic respiratory diseases and for health promotion related to chronic respiratory diseases are often absent or rudimentary.	Awareness of chronic respiratory diseases is largely insufficient.

CONTINUED ON NEXT PAGE

TABLE 1 (CONTINUED)

	Low and middle income countries	High income countries
Insufficient prevention	Exposure to risk factors for chronic respiratory diseases, including indoor air pollution, the use of solid biomass fuels and smoking, is high.	Prevention and health promotion for chronic respiratory diseases is largely insufficient. Although many risk factors predisposing people to chronic respiratory diseases are preventable, policies and legislation are still inadequate throughout the world. The Framework Convention on Tobacco Control has become an international law but there are still many countries that have yet to ratify it. As of 20 June 2007, 148 countries out of 193 WHO Member States have ratified the Convention.
	Surveillance systems and diagnostic services for work-related chronic respiratory diseases are poorly developed, and the true burden of occupational lung disease is largely unknown.	Asthma is under-diagnosed. It is often better controlled than other chronic respiratory diseases but many patients are not well controlled.
	Asthma is mostly under-diagnosed and under-treated (in particular in children), causing high morbidity and significant mortality.	COPD is largely under-diagnosed, under-treated and largely induced by smoking.
Inadequate Control	The burden of COPD is very high, in particular in the Western Pacific Region.	COPD is not regarded as a systemic disease. It is not assessed as part of chronic systemic disease surveillance (which often includes cardiovascular diseases, cancer and metabolic disorders).
	The management of conditions such as asthma and COPD emphasizes the treatment of acute episodes of exacerbations instead of care for the chronic disease and the prevention of acute episodes of exacerbations.	Work-related chronic respiratory diseases should be better identified, diagnosed and prevented.
	In some countries, additional risk factors such as altitude, parasitosis and sickle cell disease result in unique forms of chronic respiratory diseases.	In some countries, there may be additional chronic respiratory diseases associated with altitude.
	In the majority of countries, diagnostic tests (e.g. spirometry) that are required for the diagnosis and assessment of the severity of chronic respiratory diseases are not readily available, resulting in mis-assessment and under-diagnosis of chronic respiratory diseases.	Lung function testing is available in specialist practices and, in some countries, in primary care.
	Essential drugs for the treatment of chronic respiratory diseases are not available or not affordable in a large proportion of developing countries.	Drugs are usually available but are not always affordable.
	Programmes for educating health-care professionals in the care and management of patients with chronic respiratory diseases need to be strengthened.	

Public awareness of chronic respiratory disease should be increased

- Environmental barriers include tobacco smoke and other indoors pollutants, outdoor pollution, occupational exposure and nutrition. Poor nutrition is common in low and middle income countries, whereas obesity and overweight are increasing in high income countries and in urban areas of low and middle income countries (*16*).

- Availability and accessibility of drug and devices are often poor. In many countries, there is still poor accessibility to drugs (*17*,

18) despite the Bamako Initiative launched over 15 years ago (*19*). There is also a lack of resources for the diagnosis of chronic respiratory diseases in low and middle income countries.

- The potential of traditional medicine may be underestimated. In many countries, alternative and complementary medicine are commonly used. In low and middle income countries, traditional medicine is extremely important and may often be the only available therapy (*20*). Treatment with traditional medicines is usually the first step in the management of diseases, because of the beliefs of patients and taboos, the inaccessibility of health care and the high cost of drugs. In many places, traditional and modern medicine have tended to work in tandem. Because the cost of drugs is often high, the use of appropriate traditional medicine was promoted at the Fifty-fifth World Health Assembly. Unfortunately, there have as yet been no large controlled studies on the efficacy of traditional remedies in treating chronic respiratory diseases.

- There are large differences in health-care systems. Differences exist even within high income countries and are far more marked between middle and low income countries (Boxes 2 and 3).

- There is a need to put evidence into practice in low-resource settings. Gaps between evidence and practice in low and middle income countries result in ineffective treatment (*21*). There is a need to adapt guidelines into context-specific and user-friendly formats (such as algorithms, guidelines and desktop guides) (*22, 23*).

The training of health-care workers is often problematic. In most low income countries there is a lack of trained personnel, and staff turnover makes education very difficult (*21*).

Box 2 Distinct groups of people with different health-care status in low income countries

Heterogeneity of lifestyles requires a variety of health promotion, disease prevention and control strategies. In low-income countries, particular groups that need attention include:

- **People living in urban areas with a high income and with a settled and sedentary life style, including:**
  - high-income people who can afford expensive diagnostic examinations and treatments;
  - government workers who are reimbursed for diagnostic examinations and treatments;
  - industrial, agricultural or service sector workers who are reimbursed for diagnostic examinations and treatments.
- **People living in urban areas who are jobless or with limited financial resources, and people living in low income suburban or periurban areas.**
- **Poor people living in rural areas.**

Source: adapted from reference *13*.

Box 3 Major drawbacks in the organization of health-care services in low income countries

- **Inaccessibility of health-care facilities (distance, lack of facilities, or facilities not adequately staffed).**
- **Disparities in the establishment and availability of health-care facilities.**
- **Poor quality or not enough technical support.**
- **Lack qualified personnel, and no equivalence in training between the different countries.**
- **Trained personnel unlikely to stay in the same location.**

Source: adapted from reference *13*.

A vision for the future: reducing deaths and improving lives

Recent progress in public health has helped people in many parts of the world to live longer and healthier lives. The use of existing knowledge has led to major improvements in the life expectancy and quality of life of middle-aged and older people.

In *Preventing chronic diseases: a vital investment* (*1*), a global goal for preventing chronic disease is suggested to generate the sustained actions required to reduce the disease burden. The target for this proposed goal is an additional 2% annual reduction in chronic disease death rates over the decade up to 2015.

The indicators for the measurement of success towards this goal are the number of chronic disease deaths averted and the number of healthy life years gained. Most of the deaths averted from specific chronic diseases would be in low and middle income countries. It is expected that cardiovascular diseases and cancer are the diseases for which most deaths would be averted.

3. A Mechanism for Action: The Global Alliance Against Chronic Respiratory Diseases (GARD)

KEY MESSAGES

- **The Global Alliance against Chronic Respiratory Diseases (GARD) brings together national and international organizations, institutions and agencies to combat chronic respiratory diseases.**
- **GARD's goal is to reduce the global burden of chronic respiratory diseases.**
- **GARD's emphasis is on the needs of low- and middle-income countries.**

The Fifty-third World Health Assembly recognized the enormous human suffering caused by chronic diseases. It requested the WHO Director-General to give priority to the prevention and control of chronic respiratory diseases, with special emphasis on low and middle income countries and other deprived populations. The task was, in collaboration with the international community, to coordinate global partnership and alliances for resource mobilization, advocacy, capacity building and collaborative research (resolution WHA53.17, May 2000, endorsed by all WHO Member States). In order to develop a comprehensive approach for the surveillance, diagnosis, prevention and control of chronic respiratory diseases, WHO organized four consultation meetings:

- WHO Strategy for prevention and control of chronic respiratory diseases, Geneva, 11–13 January 2001 (*24*).
- Implementation of the WHO strategy for prevention and control of chronic respiratory diseases, Montpellier, 11–12 February 2002 (*25*).
- Prevention and control of chronic respiratory diseases in low and middle income African countries, Montpellier, 27–28 July 2002, and Paris, 10 June 2003 (*26*).
- Prevention and control of chronic respiratory diseases at country level: towards a global alliance against chronic respiratory diseases, Geneva, 17–19 June 2004 (*27*).

These meetings led to the formation of the Global Alliance against Chronic Respiratory Diseases (GARD) (*28*).

The Global Alliance against Chronic Respiratory Diseases (GARD) is a voluntary alliance of national and international organizations, institutions and agencies working towards the common goal of improving global lung health.

- GARD's vision: a world where all people breathe freely.
- GARD's goal: to reduce the global burden of chronic respiratory diseases.
- GARD's objective: to initiate a comprehensive approach to fight chronic respiratory diseases. This involves:

  - developing a standard way of obtaining relevant data on chronic respiratory disease risk factors;

  - encouraging countries to implement health promotion and chronic respiratory disease prevention policies;

  - recommending affordable strategies for the management of chronic respiratory diseases.

- GARD's added value: to provide a network through which collaborating parties can combine their strengths, thereby achieving results that no one partner could obtain alone; and to improve coordination between existing governmental and nongovernmental programmes, so as to avoid a duplication of efforts and the waste of resources.

- GARD's approach: to promote an integrated approach that capitalizes upon strategic synergies on prevention and control between chronic respiratory diseases and other chronic diseases; and to consider especially the needs of low and middle income countries and vulnerable populations, fostering country-specific initiatives that are tailored to local needs.

The emphasis on the needs of low- and middle-income countries is appropriate, as most cases of chronic respiratory disease occur in these countries, with communicable diseases (including HIV/AIDS) adding to the burden of chronic respiratory disease morbidity.

CHRONIC RESPIRATORY DISEASES

4. Chronic Disease Epidemics

KEY MESSAGES

- **Chronic disease epidemics take decades to become fully established.**
- **Chronic diseases often begin in childhood.**
- **Because of their slow evolution and chronic nature, chronic diseases present opportunities for prevention.**
- **Many different chronic diseases may occur in the same patient (e.g. chronic respiratory diseases, cardiovascular disease and cancer).**
- **The treatment of chronic diseases demands a long-term and systematic approach.**
- **Care for patients with chronic diseases should be an integral part of the activities of health services, alongside care for patients with acute and infectious diseases.**

Chronic respiratory diseases are a group of chronic diseases affecting the airways and the other structures of the lungs. Common chronic respiratory diseases are listed in Table 2, as they appear in ICD-10. Common symptoms of the respiratory tract are also listed in ICD-10 (Table 3).

Table 2 Common chronic respiratory diseases

Diseases	International Classification of Diseases (ICD-10)
Asthma	J44[a] –46
Bronchiectasis	A15–16[b], J44, J47, Q32–33
Chronic obstructive lung disease, including chronic obstructive pulmonary disease, bronchitis and emphysema	J40–44
Chronic rhinosinusitis	J32–33
Hypersensitivity pneumonitis	J66–67
Lung cancer and neoplasms of respiratory and intrathoracic organs	C30–39
Lung fibrosis	B90, J69, J70, J84, P27

CONTINUED ON NEXT PAGE

TABLE 2 (CONTINUED)

Diseases	International Classification of Diseases (ICD-10)
Chronic pleural diseases	C38, C45, D38, J92
Pneumoconiosis	J60–65
Pulmonary eosinophilia	J82
Pulmonary heart disease and diseases of pulmonary circulation including pulmonary embolism, pulmonary hypertension and cor pulmonale	I26–28
Rhinitis	J30–31, J45 [a]
Sarcoidosis	D86
Sleep apnea syndrome	G47

[a] Codes depicted are not exclusive of the disease listed. All codes mentioning the specific diseases were included.
[b] In patients with tuberculosis.
Source: reference *29.*

Table 3 Symptoms and signs involving the respiratory system

Respiratory symptoms	International Classification of Diseases (ICD-10)
Haemorrhage from respiratory passages ■ Epistaxis ■ Haemoptysis	R04 ■ R04.0 ■ R04.2
Cough	R05
Abnormalities of breathing ■ Dyspnoea ■ Stridor ■ Wheezing ■ Hyperventilation ■ Sneezing	R06 ■ R06.0 ■ R06.1 ■ R06.2 ■ R06.4 ■ R06.7
Pain in the throat and chest	R07
Other symptoms and signs involving the circulatory and respiratory systems ■ Asphyxia ■ Pleurisy ■ Respiratory arrest (cardiorespiratory failure) ■ Abnormal sputum	R09 ■ R09.0 ■ R09.1 ■ R09.2 ■ R09.3
Source: reference *29*.	

Hundreds of millions of people around the world suffer from preventable chronic respiratory diseases. The prevalence estimates shown in Table 4 are likely to be conservative. This report focuses on the following preventable chronic respiratory diseases and their risk factors:

- Asthma and respiratory allergies.
- Chronic obstructive pulmonary disease (COPD).

- Occupational lung diseases.
- Sleep apnea syndrome.
- Pulmonary hypertension.

Table 4 Estimates of the prevalence of preventable chronic respiratory diseases

Chronic respiratory disease	Year of estimation	Prevalence	Reference
Asthma	2004	300 million	*15*
Chronic obstructive pulmonary disease	2000	210 million	*30–32*
Allergic rhinitis	1996–2006	400 million	*33–37*
Other respiratory diseases	2006	>50 million	*38–44*
Sleep apnea syndrome	1986–2002	>100 million	*45–48*

Respiratory symptoms are among the major causes of consultation at primary health care centres. Surveys in nine countries, in 76 primary health care facilities, among which 54 (71.1%) involved medical officers and 22 (28.9%) nurses only. The number of primary health care facilities, involving 29 399 respiratory patients, showed that the proportion of patients with respiratory symptoms, among those over 5 years of age, who visited primary health care centres ranged from 8.4% to 37.0% (Table 5).

Table 5 Proportion of patients with respiratory symptoms among all patients (aged 5 years and older) who visited primary health care facilities for any reason

	Males	Females
Argentina	36.1%	32.2%
Guinea	20.6%	28.7%
Morocco (1st survey)	31.0%	21.4%
Morocco (2nd survey)	37.0%	28.7%
Nepal	17.1%	11.3%
Thailand	9.8%	8.4%

Source: reference *49*.

5. Asthma

KEY MESSAGES

- **300 million people of all ages worldwide have asthma.**
- **The prevalence of asthma has increased following changes to a modern, urban lifestyle.**
- **Globally, 250 000 people die of asthma every year.**
- **Asthma deaths are related to lack of proper treatment.**
- **Treatment for asthma is not available to all people who have asthma.**

Asthma is a chronic inflammatory disorder of the airways, usually associated with airway hyper-responsiveness and variable airflow obstruction, that is often reversible spontaneously or under treatment (*50*). Allergen sensitization is an important risk factor for asthma. Asthma is often associated with rhinitis, an inflammation of the nasal mucosa (*51*).

Prevalence

Asthma affects both children and adults. Using a conservative definition, it is estimated that as many as 300 million people of all ages and all ethnic backgrounds suffer from asthma. Two large multinational studies have assessed the prevalence of asthma around the world: the European Community Respiratory Health Survey (ECRHS) in adults (*52*) and the International Study of Asthma and Allergies in Childhood (ISAAC) in children (*33*). The world map of the prevalence of asthma (Figure 4) is based on these two studies (*15*).

Figure 4 World map of the prevalence of clinical asthma

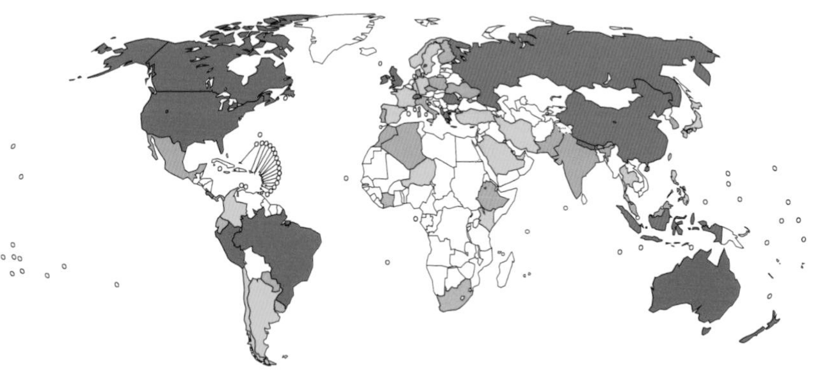

Proportion of population (%)

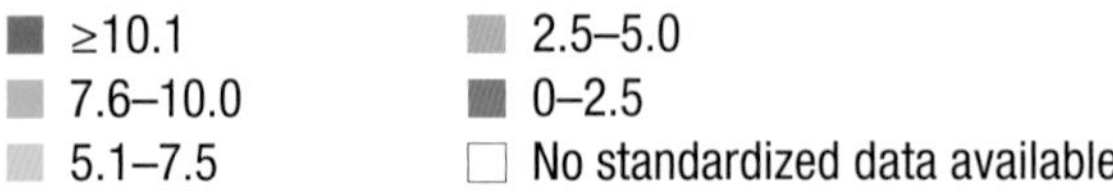

Source: reference *15*.

Trends in asthma prevalence vary between countries. For the past 40 years, the prevalence of asthma has increased in all countries in parallel with that of allergy. Asthma is still increasing worldwide as communities adopt modern lifestyles and become urbanized (*13, 53, 54*). With a projected increase in the proportion of the world's population living in urban areas, there is likely to be a marked increase in the number of people with asthma worldwide over the next two decades. It is estimated that there may be an additional 100 million people with asthma by 2025 (*15*). However, the prevalence of asthma and allergy may decrease in children in some countries with a high prevalence of the disease and the increase in the asthma epidemic may come to an end in some countries (*55–57*).

Mortality

It is estimated that asthma accounts for about 250 000 annual deaths worldwide. There are large differences between countries, and the rate of asthma deaths does not parallel prevalence (Figure 5). Mortality seems to be high in countries where access to essential drugs is low.

Figure 5 World map of asthma case fatality rates: asthma deaths per 100 000 people with asthma in the 5–34 year age group

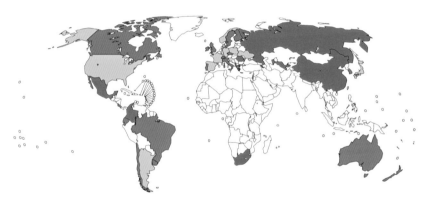

Countries shaded according to case fatality rate (per 100 000 people with asthma)

- ≥10.1
- 5.1–10.0
- 0–5.0
- No standardized data available

Source: reference *15*.

Many of the deaths are preventable, being a result of suboptimal long-term medical care and delay in obtaining help during the final attack. In many areas of the world, people with asthma do not have access to basic asthma medications and health care (*15*) (Figure 6). The countries with the highest death rates are those in which controller therapy is not available. In many countries, deaths due to asthma have declined recently as a result of better asthma management (*58*).

Morbidity

The hospitalization of patients with asthma is another measure of asthma severity, but data cannot be obtained in most low and middle income countries (*59*). In countries or regions where asthma management plans have been implemented, hospitalization rates have decreased (*58, 60*). Asthma is often severe in poor people and minorities (*61*).

Figure 6 World map of the proportion of the population with access to essential drugs

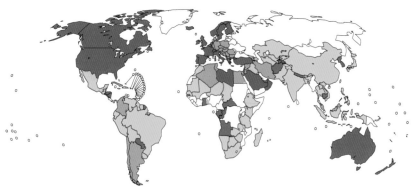

WHO Access to Essential Drugs

- <50%
- 50–80%
- 81–95%
- >95%
- No standardized data available

Source: reference *15*.

Asthma impairs school and work performance and social life (*62*). Physical quality of life is impaired by bronchial symptoms, while social life is also impaired by rhinitis co-morbidity (*63*). In 2005, in some countries of the European Union, asthma still had a major effect on patients' social life and physical activities, as well as school and work (Figure 7).

Figure 7 Effects of asthma on patients, European Union, 2005

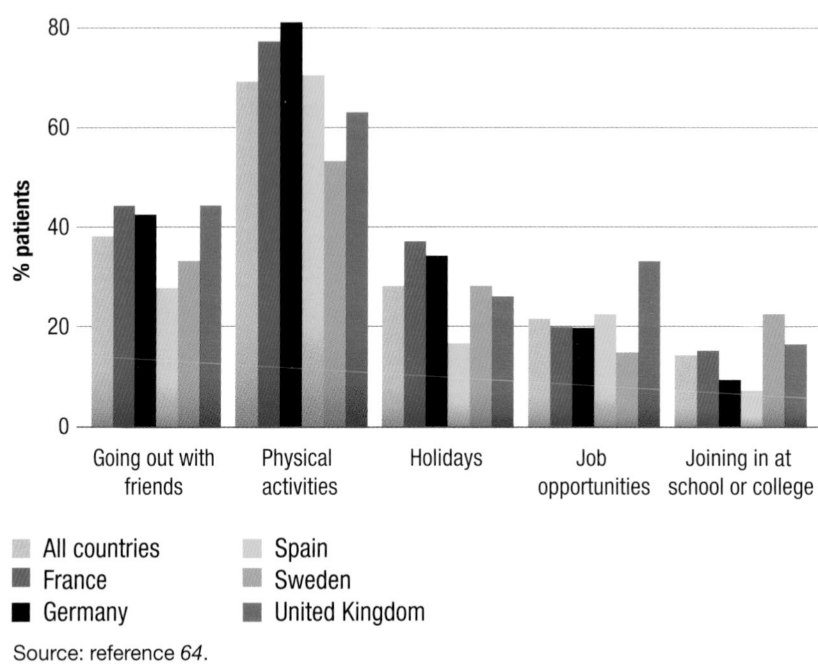

- All countries
- France
- Germany
- Spain
- Sweden
- United Kingdom

Source: reference *64*.

Childhood asthma accounts for many lost school days and may deprive the affected children of both academic achievement and social interaction, in particular in underserved populations (*65*) and minorities (*66*). Educational programmes for the self-management of asthma in children and adolescents reduce absenteeism from school and the number of days with restricted activity (*67*).

The burden of asthma assessed by disability-adjusted life years (DALYs), which ranks 22 worldwide, is similar to that of other chronic diseases such as diabetes or Alzheimer disease (Table 6).

Table 6 Disability-adjusted life years (DALYs) attributable to disorders causing the greatest burden worldwide

Rank	Disorder	Number of DALYs (x10³)
1	Lower respiratory infections	91.3
2	HIV/AIDS	84.4
3	Unipolar depressive disorders	67.2
4	Diarrhoeal diseases	61.9
5	Ischaemic heart diseases	58.6
6	Cerebrovascular disease	49.2
7	Malaria	46.5
8	Road traffic accidents	38.7
9	Tuberculosis	34.7
10	**Chronic obstructive pulmonary disease**	**27.7**
11	Congenital abnormalities	27.3
12	Hearing loss – adult onset	26.0
13	Cataracts	25.2
14	Measles	22.4
15	Violence	21.4
16	Self-inflicted injuries	20.7
17	Alcohol use disorders	20.3
18	Protein energy malnutrition	16.9
19	Falls	16.2
20	Diabetes mellitus	15.4
21	Schizophrenia	16.1
22	**Asthma**	**15.3**
23	Osteoarthritis	14.8
24	Vision loss, age-related and other	14.1
25	Cirrhosis of the liver	13.9

Source: reference *68*.

Economic costs

The economic cost of asthma is considerable both in terms of direct medical costs (such as hospital admissions and the cost of pharmaceuticals) and indirect medical costs (such as time lost from work and premature death) (*15,*

69, 70). The costs of asthma are high in severe or uncontrolled asthma (*71*). Many children with undiagnosed asthma miss school and require emergency department visits, albeit that those with a current diagnosis of asthma report more resource use (*72*). Children of low socioeconomic status are more likely to require resources because of their asthma (*73*). In low and middle income countries, childhood asthma has significant adverse effects on the child's daily activities, schooling, family life and finances (*74*).

Health-care benefits from asthma intervention programmes are clearly leading to a marked decrease in death rates and hospitalizations in high income countries (Figure 8), low and middle income countries, and deprived areas (*60, 75, 76*). In a study of 3748 low income, minority group children living in the United States, an education programme resulted in a 35% decrease in overall hospitalization rates, a 27% decrease in asthma-related visits to an emergency department and a 19% decrease in outpatient visits (*76*). However, in Finland, the asthma programme had no effect on the prevalence of the disease, which is still increasing. The number of people with asthma increased, although mortality and morbidity decreased considerably.

Figure 8 Health–care benefits of the asthma programme in Finland, 1981–1995

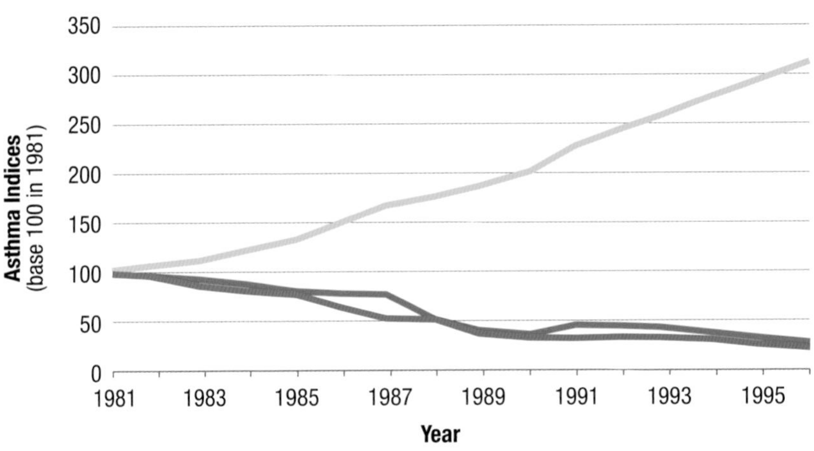

Reimbursement asthma
Hospitalization days
Death rate

Source: reference *58*.

Co-morbidities

The links between rhinitis and asthma are of importance. Epidemiological studies have consistently shown that asthma and rhinitis often co-exist in the same patients. In epidemiological studies, over 70 % of people with asthma have concomitant rhinitis (*77–79*). However, only 15 to 40% of rhinitis patients have clinically demonstrable asthma. Patients with severe persistent rhinitis have asthma more often than those with intermittent disease (*80*). Allergic and non-allergic rhinitis are associated with asthma. Although differences exist between rhinitis and asthma, upper and lower airways may be considered as a unique entity influenced by a common and probably evolving inflammatory process, which may be sustained and amplified by intertwined mechanisms (*51*).

The prevalence of rhinitis has been studied in some large epidemiological studies. According to the European Community Respiratory Health Survey (ECRHS), the prevalence of rhinitis is around 35% in Europe and Australasia (*34*). According to the International Study of Asthma and Allergy in Childhood (ISAAC), the prevalence of allergic rhinitis ranges from very low to 50% of adolescents (*81*), with an average of over 30% (*13*). The ISAAC study was carried out in the 1990s. According to more recent studies, the prevalence of allergic rhinitis has increased, in particular in countries with a low prevalence (*82–90*). In a recent study in the general population in Europe, the prevalence of allergic rhinitis was around 25% (*35, 36*). The prevalence of allergic rhinitis is increasing in developing countries. The prevalence of an IgE sensitization to aeroallergens measured by allergen specific IgE in serum or skin tests is over 40% of the population in Australia, Europe, New Zealand and the United States of America (*57, 91–93*). Most but not all of the sensitized subjects are suffering from allergic rhinitis or asthma or both.

The sequential development of allergic disease manifestations during early childhood is often referred to as the "allergy march" (*94*). Various epidemiological and birth-cohort studies have begun to elucidate the evolution of allergic disease manifestations and to identify populations at risk for disease (*95, 96*). These studies emphasize the effects of environmental factors and genetic predisposition on the allergy march. In many patients, food allergy precedes inhalant allergen allergy. In the allergy march, atopic dermatitis and asthma are linked, but atopic dermatitis does not necessarily precede asthma, whereas allergic rhinitis is a risk factor for asthma and can precede asthma (*97–99*).

In most low and middle income countries, the prevalence of active smoking in adults with asthma is about 25%. Compared to nonsmokers with asthma, active smokers have more severe asthma symptoms (*100*), an accelerated decline in lung function (*101*) and a reduced response to corticosteroid therapy (*102*). Every effort should be made to encourage individuals with asthma who smoke to stop (*103*).

6. Chronic Obstructive Pulmonary Disease

KEY MESSAGES

- **Chronic obstructive pulmonary disease (COPD) affects 210 million people.**
- **Chronic obstructive pulmonary disease was the fifth cause of death in 2002 and it is projected to be the fourth cause of mortality by 2030 (*104*).**
- **Tobacco smoking is the major risk factor, but the use indoors of solid fuels for cooking and heating also presents major risks.**
- **Strategies to reduce exposure to major risk factors are likely to have an impact on morbidity and mortality.**

Chronic obstructive pulmonary disease (COPD) is a heterogeneous disease with various clinical presentations. The basic abnormality in all patients with COPD is airflow limitation. Therefore, experts from the Global Initiative for Obstructive Lung Diseases (GOLD) have defined the disease based on spirometric criteria by using the post-bronchodilator forced expiratory volume in one second (FEV_1) and its ratio to the forced vital capacity (FVC) (*105*). The main criterion for COPD is a FEV_1/FVC ratio <70%. The terms chronic bronchitis and emphysema are no longer part of the COPD definition (Table 5) (*106, 107*).

Table 7 Definitions of chronic bronchitis, emphysema and chronic obstructive pulmonary disease

Disease	Reference	Definition	
Chronic bronchitis	108	Clinical definition	Chronic productive cough for 3 months in each of 2 consecutive years in a patient in whom other causes of productive chronic cough have been excluded.
Emphysema	108	Anatomic definition	Permanent enlargement of the airspaces distal to the terminal bronchioles, accompanied by destruction of their walls without obvious fibrosis.
Chronic obstructive pulmonary disease (COPD)	107, 109	Functional definition	Preventable and treatable disease state characterized by airflow limitation that is not fully reversible. The airflow limitation is usually progressive and associated with an abnormal inflammatory response of the lungs in response to noxious agents including cigarette smoke, biomass fuels and occupational agents. The chronic airflow limitation characteristic of COPD is caused by a mixture of small airway disease (obstructive bronchiolitis) and parenchymal destruction (emphysema). COPD is a multicomponent disease with extra-pulmonary effects.

Source: reference *110*.

Sub-classification into mild, moderate, severe and very severe disease is achieved by including various levels of FEV_1 as percentage of predicted value (Table 8) (*111*). This classification was found to correlate with pathologic findings (*112*) and the prediction for mortality (*113*).

Up to 2001, only 32 prevalence studies had been reported for COPD whereas there were hundreds for asthma and thousands for cancer or cardiovascular

Table 8 Classification of the severity of chronic obstructive pulmonary disease, based on post-bronchodilator FEV_1

Stage	Characteristics
I: Mild	FEV_1/FVC < 70% FEV_1 ≥ 80% predicted
II: Moderate	FEV_1/FVC < 70% 50% ≤ FEV_1 < 80% predicted
III: Severe	FEV_1/FVC < 70% 30% ≤ FEV_1 < 50% predicted
IV: Very severe	FEV_1/FVC < 70% FEV_1 < 30% predicted Or FEV_1 < 50% predicted plus chronic respiratory failure

FEV_1, forced expiratory volume in one second; FVC, forced vital capacity.

Respiratory failure is defined as arterial partial pressure of oxygen (PaO_2) less than 8.0 kPa (60 mmHg) with or without arterial partial pressure of CO_2 ($PaCO_2$) greater than 6.7 kPa (50 mmHg) while breathing air at sea level.

Source: reference *107*.

diseases (*114*). Fortunately, a number of initiatives are currently under way to produce new data. Some of these initiatives are presented in this report.

COPD is a major public health problem in subjects over 40 years of age and will remain a challenge for the future. It is a major cause of chronic morbidity and mortality worldwide (*107*) and is projected to rank seventh in 2030 as a worldwide burden of disease (*104*). The rise in morbidity and mortality from COPD will be most dramatic in Asian and African countries over the next two decades, mostly as a result of a progressive increase in the prevalence of smoking (*115*). Even if risk factors were avoided today, the toll of COPD would continue for several decades because of the slow development of the disease. However, a recent critical analysis of methods to estimate projections of the burden of diseases, by using extrapolation or by using risk factors, has called attention to the difficulties in having a precise definition of global trends on COPD burden (*116*).

Prevalence

Until recently, most of the information available on COPD prevalence came from high income countries. Even in these countries, data greatly underestimate the total burden of COPD because the disease is usually not diagnosed until it is clinically apparent and moderately advanced (*117*) and the definition of COPD varies between studies. An approach using the single term COPD (rather than individual coding for chronic bronchitis, emphysema and chronic airway obstruction) is favoured (*114*), although differences in prevalence rates are reported when different definitions of COPD are used (*118*).

As calculated using appropriate epidemiological methods, the prevalence of COPD is generally higher than is recognized by health authorities or administrative databases (*119*). It has been estimated to range from 4% to up to 20% in adults over 40 years of age (*120–125*), with a considerable increase by age, particularly among smokers. COPD nevertheless occurs in people aged 20–44 years (*126*) (Table 9, Figure 9). Large differences exist between countries. These are attributable to many factors, including differences in diagnostic methods, year of study, age of the population, and prevalence of main risk factors such as tobacco smoking. Overall, the prevalence estimates shown in Figure 9 and Table 9 are higher than those recorded by national registries, but they may nevertheless underestimate the real prevalence of COPD.

In the United States, in 2002, an estimated 24 million adults had COPD (*127*).

Figure 9 Prevalence rate (/100 000) of chronic obstructive pulmonary disease (COPD) in Europe

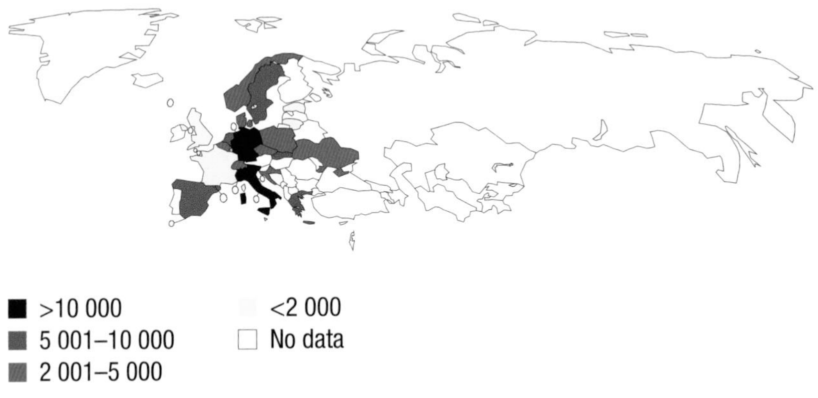

■ >10 000
■ 5 001–10 000
■ 2 001–5 000
<2 000
□ No data

Source: reference *125*.

A COPD prevalence model was used to estimate the prevalence of COPD in 12 Asian countries. The total number of moderate to severe COPD cases in the 12 countries of this region, as projected by the model, is 56.6 million with an overall prevalence rate of 6.3%. The COPD prevalence rates for the individual countries range from 3.5% (China, Hong Kong Special Administrative Region, and Singapore) to 6.7% (Viet Nam) (*158*).

In China, chronic respiratory diseases are the second leading cause of death (*32*). It is estimated that over 50% of Chinese men smoke, whereas smoking rates among women are lower in this country (*159*). The prevalence of COPD in men and women in China is not very different (*160*), which points to the importance of risk factors other than smoking in causing COPD in Chinese women. A recent study found a prevalence of physician-diagnosed COPD of 5.9% in the adult population (*160*).

In India, a study collecting data without spirometry assessment suggested that 12 million people were affected by COPD (*161*). Recent studies from the same authors (*162, 163*) show a prevalence of respiratory symptoms in 6%–7% of non-smokers and up to 14% of smokers. In a recent study in southern India, the prevalence rate of COPD in adults was around 7%.

The Burden of Obstructive Lung Disease (BOLD) study is currently being carried out in different parts of the world including low and middle income countries (*164*). This very important study compares the prevalence and burden of COPD across the world using the same protocol, including the BOLD questionnaire and spirometry. Some results are already available and show

Table 9 Prevalence estimates of chronic obstructive pulmonary disease (COPD) by diagnostic approach

Country	Reference	Year	Diagnostic criteria	Age (years)	COPD prevalence (%)		
					Overall	Males	Females
Spirometry–based diagnosis							
Denmark	*(128)*	1989	$FEV_1/FVC<70\%$, $FEV_1<60\%$ predicted	20–90	3.7		
England	*(129)*	1999	$FEV_1<5^{th}$ percentile + reversibility	60–75	9.9		
Finland	*(130)*	1994	Clinical examination + spirometry	≥ 65		12.5	3.0
	(131)	2000	Clinical examination + spirometry	≥ 30		22.1	7.2
			$FEV_1/FVC<70\%$, $FEV_1<60\%$ predicted			11.0	5.2
Italy	*(120)*	2000	ERS spirometric criteria	≥ 25	11.0	12.5	11.8
Norway	*(132)*	1979	Clinical examination + spirometry	16–69	4.1	3.7	4.6
	(133)	1991	Symptoms + spirometry	18–70	5.4	5.6	5.2
			$FEV_1/FVC<70\%$, $FEV_1<80\%$ predicted		4.5	4.8	4.2
Spain	*(134)*	1998	$FEV_1/FVC<70\%$, $FEV_1<80\%$ predicted	40–60		6.8	
	(135)	2000	ERS spirometric criteria + reversibility	40–69	9.1	14.3	3.9
USA	*(136)*	1971	$FEV_1/FVC<60\%$	20–69		13.0	2.0
	(137)	2000	$FEV_1/FVC<70\%$, $FEV_1<80\%$ predicted	≥ 17	6.8		
Symptom-based diagnosis (chronic bronchitis)							
Australia	*(138)*	1968	MRC criteria	≥ 21		9.0	3.0
Brazil	*(139, 140)*	1994-1995	MRC criteria	≥ 40	12.7	17.9	9.1
Denmark	*(128)*	1989	Daily phlegm ≥ 3 months for ≥ 1 year	20–90	10.1	12.5	8.2
England	*(141)*	1989	MRC criteria	40–74		16.7	7.1
Iceland	*(142)*	1999	ATS criteria	50–80		7.1	16.7
India	*(143)*	1994	MRC criteria	≥ 15	7.7	7.6	7.8
Nepal	*(144)*	1984	MRC criteria	≥ 20	18.3	17.6	18.9
Area comprising the state of Zimbabwe	*(145)*	1978	MRC criteria	>20	1.1	1.2	1.5
Spain	*(134)*	1998	ECSC criteria	40–60		9.2	
USA	*(135)*	1971	MRC criteria	20–69		17.0	10.0
	(146)	1977	Cough and phlegm ≥ 3 months	20–74		17	6

CONTINUED ON NEXT PAGE

TABLE 9 (CONTINUED)

Country	Reference	Year	Diagnostic criteria	Age (years)	COPD prevalence (%)		
					Overall	Males	Females
Multiple	*(147)*	1997	3 criteria based on symptoms and history	50–69		1.2-12.9	
Multiple	*(148)*	2001	MRC criteria	20–44	3.2	3.7	2.8
Patient-reported disease							
	(149)	2000	Physician diagnosed	35–44		1.8	3.5
				45–54		1.5	3.6
Canada				55–64		5.0	4.5
	(150)	1999	Physician diagnosed	≥ 55	5.7	6.3	5.2
England	*(141)*		Patient report (chronic bronchitis)	40–74		3.9	2.1
Estonia	*(151)*	2001	Physician diagnosed (chronic bronchitis)	54–64	10.7	9.3	11.5
Finland	*(152)*	1999	Physician diagnosed	20–69	3.7		
Hong Kong SAR	*(153)*	1995	Patient report of disease	≥ 70	8.0	10.7	5.5
Sweden	*(154)*	1991	Physician diagnosed	35–66	4.1	4.7	4.0
	(155)	1998	Physician diagnosed	20–59	3.7		
USA	*(156)*	1975	Patient report (chronic bronchitis)	All ages	6.6		
	(157)	1996	Patient report (chronic bronchitis)	All ages	5.4		

[a] MRC, Medical Research Council ; ATS, American Thoracic Society ; ECSC, European Commission for Steel and Coal.
Source: reference *121*.

that the prevalence of COPD is far higher than is recorded. In Guangdong, China (*165*), the prevalence of COPD is 9.4% and it is higher in the rural area than in the urban area suggesting a synergic effect of smoking and biomass burning. In Latin America (*166*), the *Proyecto Latinoamericano de Investigacion en Obstruccion Pulmonar* (the PLATINO Project) (*167, 168*) showed that COPD prevalence was over 10% in subjects older than 40 years of age (Table 10). The results shown in Table 10 were obtained using the BOLD method (*164*). These results indicate that the prevalence of COPD is higher than previously reported, and that women who do not smoke can be affected by COPD. Most patients have mild COPD. However, the concomitant diagnosis of asthma, chronic bronchitis or emphysema is common among COPD patients from the general population, particularly in adults aged over 50 years (*123, 169*). It is important to make the distinction between asthma and COPD, even in older patients because their optimal management must be based on distinctively different approaches (*27, 50, 106*).

Smoking is a major risk factor in men (*170*). In non-smoking women, unexpectedly, the prevalence of COPD is also high in high income countries, as well as in low and middle income countries. In low and middle income countries, COPD in women may be associated with biomass burning.

Table 10 Prevalence of chronic obstructive pulmonary disease (COPD) in Latin America: results of the PLATINO study

		Sao Paulo Brazil	Santiago Chile	Mexico city Mexico	Montevideo Uruguay	Caracas Venezuela
Sex	Men	18.0%	23.3%	11.0%	27.1%	15.7%
	Women	14.0%	12.8%	5.6%	14.5%	10.2%
Age	40–49 years	8.4%	7.1%	2.2%	5.1%	5.4%
	50–51 years	16.2%	13.0%	4.5%	12.7%	9.8%
	≥ 60 years	25.7%	30.3%	18.4%	21.2%	23.4%
COPD[a] stage	Stage 0	25.3%	33.6%	23.2%	19.1%	23.1%
	Stage I	10.1%	11.0%	5.2%	12.5%	6.4%
	Stage II	4.6%	4.9%	1.9%	6.4%	4.9%
	Stage III	0.9%	0.7%	0.5%	0.6%	0.7%
	Stage IV	0.2%	0.3%	0.2%	0.1%	0.1%
Education (years)	0–2	22.1%	33.3%	11.3%	29.4%	16.2%
	3–4	16.3%	21.4%	12.1%	23.5%	13.7%
	5–8	14.4%	17.7%	6.1%	21.4%	12.0%
	≥ 9	10.4%	13.6%	6.0%	15.2%	10.6%
Smoking	Never	12.5%	15.9%	6.2%	15.3%	6.6%
	0–9.9 pack–years	12.8%	13.9%	6.3%	14.3%	8.1%
	10–19.9 pack–years	15.3%	15.5%	15.7%	14.7%	15.3%
	≥ 20 pack–years	24.6%	30.8%	15.4%	32.0%	24.8%

[a] COPD was defined as post-bronchodilator $FEV_1/FVC<70\%$.
Source: reference *168*.

Mortality

Mortality data are rarely available. When available, they usually underestimate COPD as a cause of death by around 50% (*171, 172*). Moreover, there may be misuses of mortality data such as attributing death to cor pulmonale when this condition was caused by COPD (*173*). The proportion of deaths from various diseases, as reported in the United States, is shown in Figure 10 (*174*). In Europe, large differences exist and they are likely to be attributable to variations in reporting and risk factors (Figure 11).

Figure 10 Deaths from lung diseases in the United States in 2001

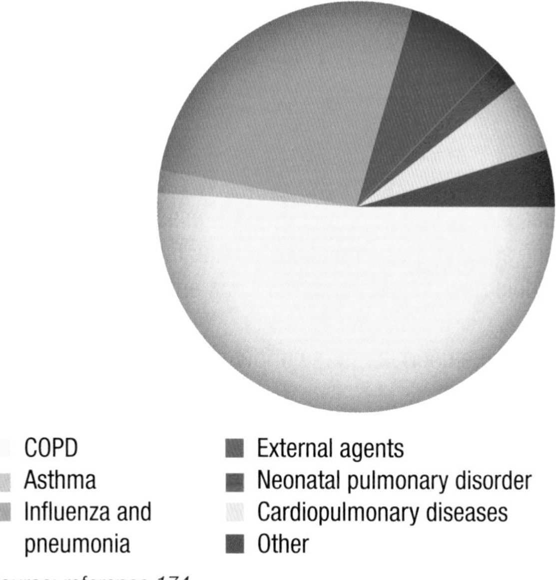

Source: reference *174*.

Figure 11 Mortality rate (/100 000) attributable to chronic obstructive pulmonary disease (COPD) in Europe

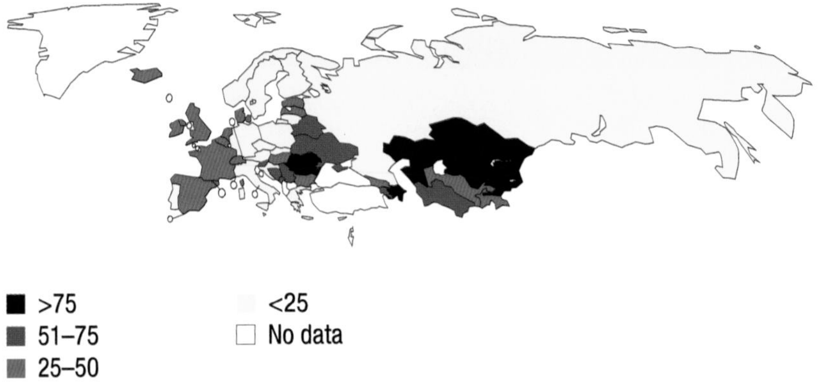

Source: reference *125*.

Deaths attributable to COPD have increased sharply in countries where data are available. According to WHO, COPD will move from fifth leading cause of death in 2002, to fourth place in the rank projected to 2030 worldwide (*104*). In high income countries, COPD is the major chronic disease for which deaths are increasing. In the USA, death rates for COPD have doubled between 1970 and 2002 (*175*) (Figure 12). There is a perception that COPD affects more males than females; however, 50.3% of the deaths attributable to COPD in 2000 in the USA were among women (*176*). In Latin America, COPD deaths have increased by 65.0% in the last decade (*166*). Treatment interventions were found to reduce COPD mortality (*177*).

Figure 12 Trends in age-standardized death rates for the six leading causes in the United States, 1970 to 2020

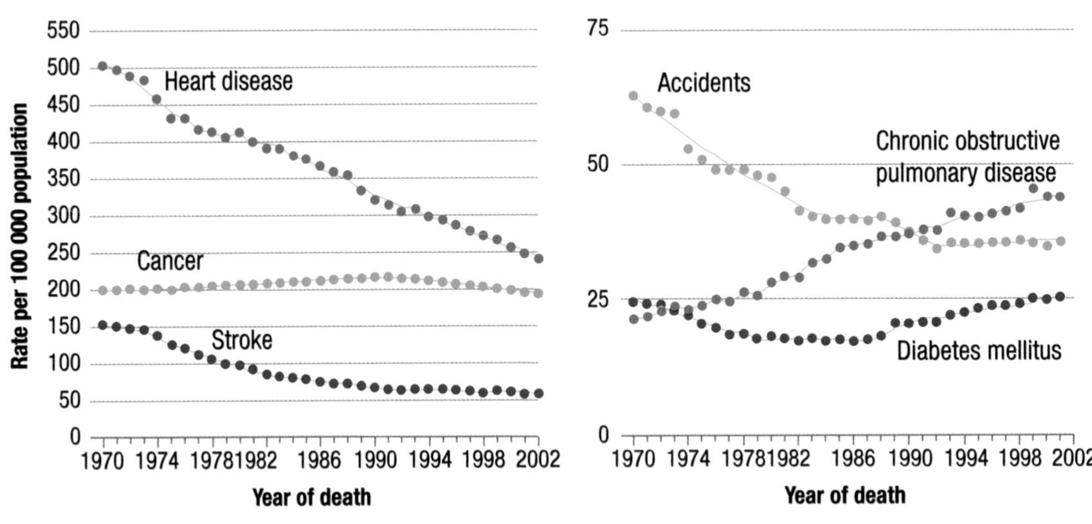

Source: reference *175*.

Morbidity

COPD is a major cause of chronic morbidity worldwide (*107, 178*). It is projected that it will rank seventh in 2030 as a worldwide burden of disease (*104*) (Table 11).

Table 11 Changes in rankings for 15 leading causes of DALYs, 2002 and 2030

Category	Disease or injury	2002 Rank	2030 Ranks	Change in Ranks
Within top 15	Perinatal conditions	1	5	-4
	Lower respiratory infections	2	8	-6
	HIV/AIDS	3	1	+2
	Unipolar depressive disorders	4	2	+2
	Diarrhoeal diseases	5	12	-7
	Ischaemic heart disease	6	3	+3
	Cerebrovascular disease	7	6	+1
	Road traffic accidents	8	4	+4
	Malaria	9	15	-6
	Tuberculosis	10	25	-15
	COPD	11	7	+4
	Congenital anomalies	12	20	-8
	Hearing loss, adult onset	13	9	+4
	Cataracts	14	10	+4
	Violence	15	13	+2
Outside top 15	Self-inflicted injuries	17	14	+3
	Diabetes mellitus	20	11	+9

Source: reference *104*.

COPD severely impairs quality of life (*179, 180*). There are multiple generic and disease-specific instruments that can be used to measure health-related quality of life (HRQOL), each incorporating various aspects of physical, psychological and social function (*181*). The association between HRQOL and lung function is usually weak, whereas it is greater with COPD co-morbidities (*182*). Exacerbations lead to substantial reductions in HRQOL, both in physical as well as other domains (*183*). HRQOL usually improves on resolution of the exacerbation (*181*).

Acute exacerbations of COPD are a common cause of morbidity and mortality. There is no universally accepted definition of an exacerbation of COPD (*184*). Most definitions use an increase in symptoms requiring increased treatment. The common etiological factors are bacterial or viral infections and air pollutants. There are no data on the frequency, severity and duration of exacerbations in COPD. Exacerbations of COPD adversely affect the natural history of COPD (*185*). Hospitalizations attributable to COPD are common and their frequency is recognized as a prognostic marker (*186*). The European Respiratory Society (ERS) white book states that the number of hospitalizations for COPD in 1993 in Germany was 125 000, in Italy 40 000, and in the United Kingdom 73 000 (*125*). Hospitalizations attributable to COPD are sharply increasing in most countries.

Economic costs

The economic burden of COPD is considerable and will continue to grow as the number of elderly people continues to increase (*187*). Data are, however, limited and available only for high income countries (Table 12). BOLD is developing a health economic model to estimate the future burden of COPD and to assess the cost–effectiveness of an intervention.

Table 12 Comparison of the costs associated with chronic obstructive pulmonary disease (COPD) in different countries

Country	Reference	Year of publication	Costs	Cost per patient per year	Global costs per year (in millions)
Spain	*(188)*	1992		€ 959	Direct: € 319 Indirect: € 451
USA	*(189)*	2000	Direct	Stage I: US$ 1681 Stage II: US$ 5037 Stage III: US$ 10 812	
Sweden	*(190)*	2000	Direct and indirect		Direct: € 109 Indirect: € 541
USA	*(191)*	2000	Direct	emphysema: US$ 1341 chronic bronchitis: US$ 816	US$ 14 500
Netherlands	*(192)*	1999	Direct	US$ 876	
Italy	*(193)*	2002	Direct	Stage I: € 151 Stage II: € 3001 Stage III: € 3912	
Sweden	*(194)*	2002	Direct and indirect	US$ 12 984	
Spain	*(195)*	2003	Direct	Stage I: € 1185 Stage II: € 1640 Stage III: € 2333	€ 427
Spain	*(196)*	2004	Direct	€ 909	€ 239
USA	*(197)*	2005	Direct and indirect		US$ 32 000

Source: reference *114*.

In the United States, in 2000, total annual costs were in excess of US$ 32 billion (*197*). The majority of patients using health-care resources are those with moderate to severe disease, with this group responsible for up to 70% of the total medical expenditure in the United States (*176*). Hospitalizations for acute exacerbation of COPD are the major contributor to the annual cost. COPD is the most expensive of the chronic diseases found in elderly patients. COPD is the fourth most common diagnosis cited on discharge for all hospitalized elderly people and the most common diagnosis for those aged 65 to 74 years (*197*). Direct costs increase with COPD severity, as assessed by FEV_1 values (*198*) (Figure 13).

In the European Union, among respiratory diseases, COPD is the leading cause of work days lost (*125*).

Figure 13 Costs for chronic obstructive pulmonary disease (COPD) in the United States, by severity as assessed using FEV_1 values

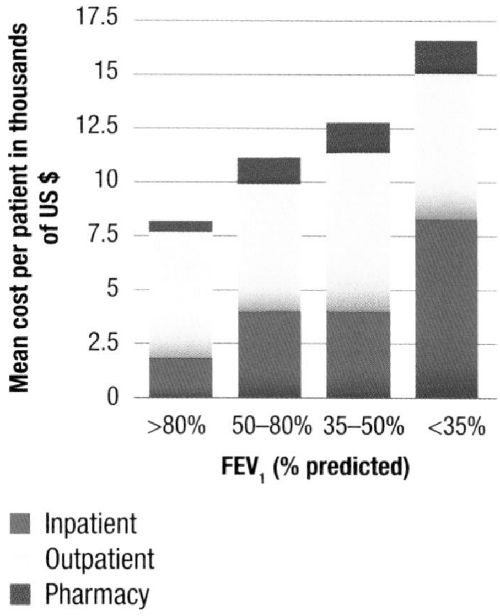

Source: reference *198*.

COPD in women

The effect of COPD on women is not sufficiently studied, but there appear to be sex differences in the prevalence, severity, risk factors (*199, 200*) and death rates (Figure 14).

In the NAHNES III study carried out among 13 995 non-smokers, 4.7 ± 0.3% had mild COPD (age, 60.9 ± 1.3 years) and were mostly female (82.5%), while 1.9 ± 0.3% had moderate-to-severe COPD (age 39.3 ± 1.3 years) and were mostly male (88.1%). Few non-smokers with COPD (12.1 ± 2.4%) had

Figure 14 Age–adjusted death rates for chronic obstructive pulmonary disease (COPD) in males and females aged 35–74 years

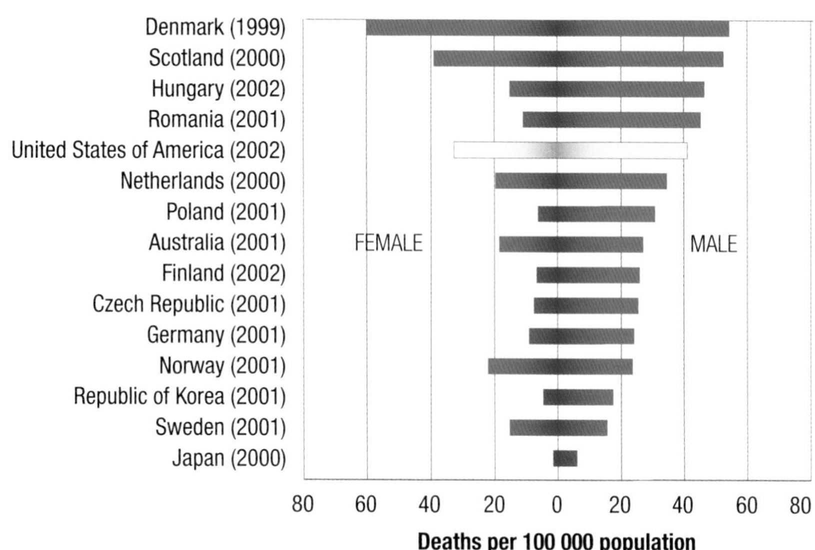

Source: reference *202*.

a previous diagnosis of chronic bronchitis or emphysema. Similar data have been found in Japan (*124*).

It is possible that the level of FEV_1 in smokers has a different effect in men and women since, in the Euroscop study, reduced baseline FEV_1 was associated with respiratory symptoms in men but not in women (*201*).

Sex differences in hyper-responsiveness were first noted in the Lung Health Study (*203*). Women are more predisposed to suffer the adverse respiratory consequences of tobacco smoking, with the development of COPD at an earlier age and with a greater degree of lung function impairment for a given amount of tobacco exposure (*204–206*). Women may benefit most from smoking cessation (*206, 207*). Conversely, reduction in smoking behaviour has been more pronounced in men than women.

Co-morbidities

COPD is a multi-component and systemic disease (*208, 209*). The components affect both the lungs and organs outside the lungs – the so-called systemic effects of COPD (*210–212*) – and can be of either a structural (including airway remodelling, emphysema, skeletal muscle wasting or osteoporosis) or functional nature (inflammation, apoptosis, senescence). Furthermore, these components are interdependent in a closely linked vicious cycle.

Even allowing for common etiological factors, a link has been identified between COPD and other systemic diseases (*213*), such as cardiovascular disease (*214*), diabetes (*215*), osteoporosis (*216*) and possibly peptic ulcer.

COPD and other disorders associated with reduced lung function are strong risk factors for cardiovascular hospitalizations and deaths, independent of smoking (*214, 217, 218*). Studies suggest that cardiovascular risk should be monitored and treated with particular care in any adult with COPD (219) and that COPD and other co-morbidities should be carefully considered in patients with chronic heart failure (*220*).

COPD and lung cancer are common in the same patients (*221*). Although other risk factors for lung cancer exist, smoking is the major risk factor. The presence of moderate or severe obstructive lung disease is a significant predictor of lung cancer in the long term (*222*). The screening for lung cancer in patients at risk is, however, still a matter of debate (*223*).

7. Obstructive Sleep Apnea Syndrome

KEY MESSAGES

- **Obstructive sleep apnea syndrome is the most common organic sleep disorder.**
- **It may affect children and adults, and result in excessive daytime somnolence and poor performance.**
- **It has been associated with increased frequency of accidents and arterial hypertension.**

Snoring and sleep apnea are common disorders that affect both men and women. The prevalence of snoring and obstructive sleep apnea syndrome increases with age, with a peak between the ages of 55 to 60 years (45–48). Women start to snore later in life, with an increased prevalence after menopause.

Obstructive sleep apnea syndrome is a clinical disorder marked by recurring episodes of upper airway obstruction that lead to markedly reduced (hypopnea) or absent (apnea) airflow at the nose or mouth. These episodes are usually accompanied by loud snoring and hypoxemia, and are typically terminated by brief micro-arousals, which result in sleep fragmentation (*224*). Patients with obstructive sleep apnea syndrome are typically unaware of such arousals, but the resulting deterioration in sleep quality contributes greatly to excessive daytime sleepiness. Most obstructive sleep apnea syndrome patients have no detectable respiratory abnormality while awake.

Prevalence

The prevalence of obstructive sleep apnea syndrome has been extensively studied in recent decades and has been variously estimated at between 1% and over 6% of the adult population (*225–229*). The Wisconsin cohort study, which studied 1069 employed men and women between 30 and 60 years of age by means of full polysomnography (*225*) found that 9% of women and 24% of men had an apnea index greater than 5 per hour but this estimate of prevalence fell to 2% of women and 4% of men when an apnea index >5 was combined with symptomatic daytime sleepiness. These findings underline the importance of not viewing obstructive sleep apnea syndrome in terms of sleep-related breathing disturbances alone. In a Spanish community study, 6.5% of males met the minimal diagnostic criteria for obstructive sleep apnea syndrome with an apnea-hypopnea index > 5 combined with daytime sleepiness (*226*). In Hong Kong Special Administrative Region, China, the prevalence of symptomatic obstructive sleep apnea syndrome is over 4% of men and over 2% of women ranging in age from 30 to 60 years (*230, 231*). A summary of prevalence from other major epidemiological studies is provided in Table 13.

The male to female ratio of obstructive sleep apnea syndrome is about two to one. This greater prevalence in males is still poorly understood. However, sex-specific hormones may play a role, with androgens promoting upper airway collapsibility (*232*), while progesterone, in contrast, seems to lead to an augmented ventilatory response. It has long been recognized that sleep apnea is very common in elderly people but the clinical significance of this

Table 13 Prevalence of obstructive sleep apnea syndrome

Country and reference	Population subjects	Age (years)	Criteria	Prevalence (%)
USA *(225)*	352 men 250 women	30–60 30–60	Hypersomnia and RDI>5	4.0 (M) 2.0 (F)
Spain *(226)*	2148 1050 men 1098 women	30–70	AHI >5 plus symptoms	6.5 (M) 3 (F)
USA *(227)*	4364 men Subsample: 741	20–100	AHI>10 plus daytime symptoms	3.3 45–64 years: 4.7
United Kingdom *(228)*	893 men	35–65	ODI_4 >20, symptomatic ODI_4>10 ODI_4>5	0.3 1.0 4.6
Australia *(229)*	294 men	40–65	RDI>10 Subjective EDS and RDI>5	10.0 3.0

RDI, respiratory disturbance index; AHI, apnea/hypopnea index; ODI_4, oxygen desaturation > 4%; EDS, excessive daytime sleepiness; M, males; F, females.

finding remains unclear (*233, 234*). While many of these subjects are otherwise asymptomatic for obstructive sleep apnea syndrome, there is evidence that sleep apnea in elderly people has an adverse prognosis (*234*).

Children may develop a sleep apnea syndrome similar to that seen in adults, and various epidemiological reports suggest a relatively high prevalence, although somewhat less than in adults (*235, 236*). The etiology of obstructive sleep apnea syndrome in children differs from the etiology in adults in that adenotonsillar hypertrophy is the most common cause of the disorder, although the increasing prevalence of obesity among children in recent years represents an important contributing factor in many cases. Many children with obstructive sleep apnea syndrome can be helped by tonsillectomy.

Morbidity and mortality

The principal physical morbidity and mortality of obstructive sleep apnea syndrome relates to the cardiovascular system. However, there is a high prevalence of other cardiovascular risk factors in patients with obstructive sleep apnea syndrome, which makes the identification of an independent contribution from obstructive sleep apnea syndrome to cardiovascular disease more difficult (*237*). The Sleep Heart Health Study, which includes over 6000 volunteer subjects undergoing in-home polysomnography, identified a modest independent association with hypertension (odds ratio 1.37), increasing with greater severity of the disease (*238*). The Wisconsin Sleep Cohort study identified an even stronger correlation with an odds ratio of 3.1 (*239*). There is also growing evidence of an independent link between obstructive sleep apnea syndrome to other cardiovascular diseases. In the Sleep Heart Health Study cohort, obstructive sleep apnea syndrome emerged as an independent risk factor for congestive cardiac failure (odds ratio 2.2), cerebrovascular disease (odds ratio 1.58) and coronary artery disease (odds ratio 1.27) (*240*). Furthermore, effective continuous positive airway pressure therapy decreases cardiovascular morbidity and mortality, as demonstrated in long-term cardiovascular outcome studies (*241–243*).

Economic costs

There is evidence that, prior to diagnosis, patients with obstructive sleep apnea syndrome incur higher health-care costs than matched control subjects (*244–247*). One study reported that obstructive sleep apnea syndrome patients used more than twice as many healthcare services in the 10-year period prior to diagnosis compared to controls (*244*), and the excess cost compared to control subjects was in the region of 4265 Canadian dollars per patient. Furthermore, the same group reported a significant reduction in health-care costs in the two-year period after introduction of continuous positive airway pressure therapy, compared to the 5-year period before diagnosis and also compared to matched controls during the same 7-year period of follow-up (*246*). Another study (*247*) reported an annual health-care use cost of US$ 2720 for obstructive sleep apnea syndrome patients prior to diagnosis, compared to US$ 1384 among matched control subjects.

The economic costs of obstructive sleep apnea syndrome should also be placed in the context of the potential impact of untreated disease on society. There is now clear evidence of an increased risk of road traffic accidents in untreated patients with obstructive sleep apnea syndrome. Various studies have demonstrated an increase in accident rate to between 3 and 7 times that of the general population among untreated obstructive sleep apnea syndrome patients; these rates fall to normal levels after successful therapy with continuous positive airway pressure (*248–250*).

A further aspect of the economic cost of obstructive sleep apnea syndrome relates to diagnosis and treatment. The traditional approach to diagnosis has been the demonstration of the disorder through overnight sleep studies in a dedicated sleep laboratory (*251*). These studies are, however, resource intensive. Increasing emphasis is thus being placed on limited diagnostic techniques that focus on cardio-respiratory variables and are suitable for home-based studies (*252*). The cost of treatment with continuous positive airway pressure is relatively modest (*253*) – involving the provision of a device with a lifespan of at least 5 years – and compares favourably with the cost of treatment for other chronic respiratory disorders such as asthma and chronic obstructive pulmonary disease.

Co-morbidities

Obstructive sleep apnea syndrome is associated with many adverse sequelae, both behavioural and physical. Behavioural consequences include daytime sleepiness, impaired concentration and neuropsychological dysfunction (*254, 255*) while physical consequences include cardiovascular disorders, particularly hypertension (*238–241, 256*). However, the excessive daytime sleepiness and associated behavioural consequences of obstructive sleep apnea syndrome are reversible with effective treatment, and there is emerging evidence that cardiovascular complications also benefit from therapy (*242, 243, 257*).

8. Pulmonary Hypertension

KEY MESSAGES

- **Pulmonary hypertension may be primary, or a consequence of various conditions, such as chronic obstructive pulmonary disease, pulmonary fibrosis, sickle cell disease and schistosomiasis.**
- **It is often associated with a poor prognosis.**
- **Interventions to control risk factors and treat pulmonary hypertension may reduce the burden of the disease.**

Pulmonary hypertension is defined as a mean pulmonary artery pressure above 25 mm Hg (*258*). If untreated, this condition has a poor prognosis.

Idiopathic pulmonary arterial hypertension, also known as primary pulmonary hypertension, is rare and has an estimated prevalence of 6 per million in France. Pulmonary arterial hypertension associated with other conditions such as systemic sclerosis, congenital heart diseases, portal hypertension and HIV infection has a cumulated prevalence of around 15 per million (*259*). Although it is not a common disease, pulmonary hypertension affects millions of patients around the world.

Several major risk factors of pulmonary hypertension have been identified (Figure15). Pulmonary hypertension and cor pulmonale may complicate many advanced pulmonary conditions including COPD (*260, 261*), bronchiectasis, cystic fibrosis, or lung fibrosis. When present, pulmonary hypertension directly contributes to disability and early mortality, causing a heavy burden worldwide.

Figure 15 Countries where schistosomiasis is prevalent

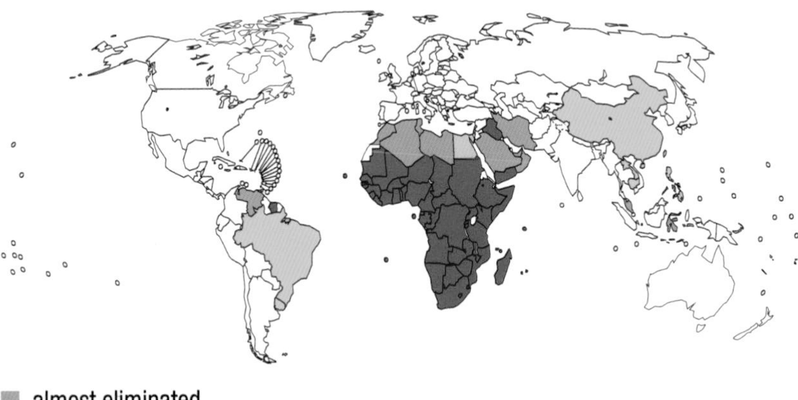

- almost eliminated
- ongoing large–scale control
- limited or no control

Source: reference *267*.

Pulmonary hypertension may affect a substantial proportion of highlanders in many countries, causing a large burden in Bolivia and other Andean countries, as well as in Kyrgyzstan, China and other Himalayan countries (*44, 262, 263*).

Pulmonary hypertension is a major cause of disability and mortality in patients with hepatosplenic forms of schistosomiasis, causing a heavy burden in Brazil, Egypt, South-East Asia and sub-Saharan Africa (*40, 264, 265*). It is estimated that up to 20% of patients with schistosomiasis (Figure 15) may suffer from pulmonary hypertension. Many aspects of morbidity attributable to schistosomiasis are expected to change after schistosomiasis is controlled (*266*). Some aspects are expected to change quickly (worm burden, Salmonella bacteraemia, hepatosplenic schistosomiasis in children), whereas others will persist for years (pulmonary hypertension, glomerulonephritis, neuroschistosomiasis).

Pulmonary hypertension is a major cause of disability and mortality in patients with sickle cell disease and thalassaemia, causing a substantial burden in Africa and in people of African origin worldwide, as well as in people from Mediterranean countries (*268*). In adult patients with sickle cell disease, although the rise in pulmonary arterial pressure is mild, the associated morbidity and mortality are high, and pulmonary hypertension is emerging as the major independent risk factor for death (*42*).

Patients with tuberculosis, HIV infection, liver cirrhosis, autoimmune diseases, congenital heart diseases and sarcoidosis are also at risk for pulmonary hypertension (*259*).

After an acute pulmonary embolism, up to 3% of patients may develop chronic thrombo-embolic pulmonary disease. This may lead to severe chronic thrombo-embolic pulmonary hypertension, a condition that can be cured by means of surgical thrombo-endarterectomy.

Obesity has been associated with various forms of pulmonary hypertension, mainly attributable to associated risk factors such as appetite suppressant intake, hypoxemia, left heart disease and thrombo-embolic disease (*269*).

RISK FACTORS FOR CHRONIC RESPIRATORY DISEASES

9. Causes and Consequences of Chronic Respiratory Diseases

KEY MESSAGES

- **Many risk factors for chronic respiratory diseases have been identified and can be prevented.**
- **Major risk factors include:**

  tobacco smoke
  second hand tobacco smoke
  other indoor air pollutants
  outdoor air pollutants
  allergens
  occupational agents.

- **Possible risk factors include:**

  diet and nutrition
  post infectious chronic respiratory diseases.

Many risk factors of chronic respiratory diseases among those of chronic diseases have been identified (Table 14).

Table 14 Risk factors for chronic respiratory diseases among those of chronic diseases

Each year:

- 7.1 million people die as a result of raised blood pressure
- 4.9 million people die as a result of tobacco use
- 4.4 million people die as a result of raised cholesterol levels
- 2.7 million people die as a result of low fruit and vegetable consumption
- 2.6 million people die as a result of being overweight or obese
- 1.9 million people die as a result of physical inactivity
- 1.6 million people die as a result of being exposed to solid fuels.[a]

[a] Includes acute respiratory infections and chronic respiratory diseases.
Source: references 1 and 270.

The causes of the chronic respiratory diseases are well known (Figure 16). The most important modifiable risk factors are: tobacco use, other exposures

Figure 16 Causes of chronic respiratory diseases

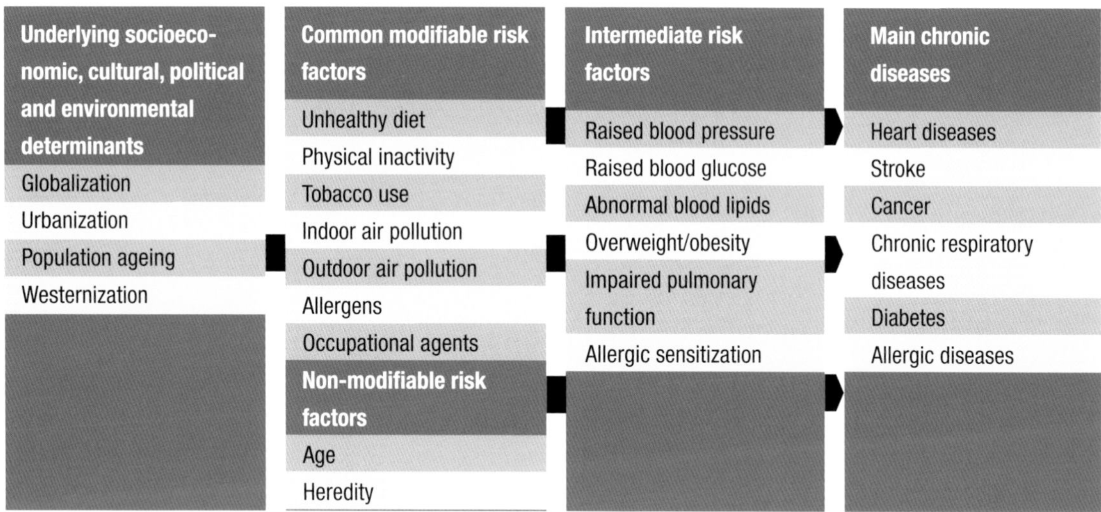

Source: reference *1*.

to indoor and outdoor air pollutants, allergens, occupational exposure, and to a lesser extent than for other chronic diseases, unhealthy diet, obesity and overweight intake and physical inactivity.

Preventable risk factors

In attempting to reduce risks to health, the first steps are to quantify the health risks and to assess their distribution. The risk factors for chronic respiratory diseases are presented in Tables 15 and 16.

Table 15 Disability-adjusted life years (DALYs) (in millions) attributable to various risk factors, by level of socioeconomic development and sex, 2000

	High mortality developing country		Low mortality developing country		Developed country	
	Males	Females	Males	Females	Males	Females
Total DALYs	421	412	223	185	118	97
	(% of total)	(% of total)	(% of total)	(% of total)	(% of total)	(% of total)
Tobacco	3.4	0.6	6.2	1.3	17.1	6.2
Indoor smoke from solid fuels	3.7	3.6	1.5	2.3	0.2	0.3
Urban air pollution	0.4	0.3	1.0	0.9	0.6	0.5
Occupational airborne particulates	0.1	<0.1	0.87	0.1	0.4	0.1

Source: reference *7*.

Risk accumulation with age

Populations are ageing in most low and middle income countries, against a background of many unsolved infrastructural problems. In the 1960s, people

Table 16 Mortality (in millions) attributable to various risk factors, by level of socioeconomic development and sex, 2000

	High mortality developing country		Low mortality developing country		Developed country	
	Males	Females	Males	Females	Males	Females
Total deaths	13.8	12.7	8.6	7.4	6.9	6.6
	(% of total)	(% of total)	(% of total)	(% of total)	(% of total)	(% of total)
Tobacco	7.5	1.5	12.2	2.9	26.3	9.3
Indoor smoke from solid fuels	3.6	4.3	1.9	5.4	0.1	0.2
Urban air pollution	0.9	0.8	2.5	2.9	1.1	1.2
Occupational airborne particulate	0.3	<0.1	1.6	0.2	0.6	0.1

Source: reference *7*.

aged 60 years and over constituted only a small minority, but their number is increasing rapidly. Ageing is a process associated with chronic and disabling diseases (Figure 17). Chronic respiratory diseases are among the most frequent and severe of all, also in the elderly.

In low and middle income countries, those who spent a large part of their lives in an urban setting tended to have unhealthier lifestyles and therefore a higher risk of chronic diseases compared with their less urbanized counterparts. An exception to this rule may arise from exposure to indoor air pollution in rural areas where solid fuels are used for cooking and heating.

Figure 17 Risk accumulation: a life approach to chronic diseases

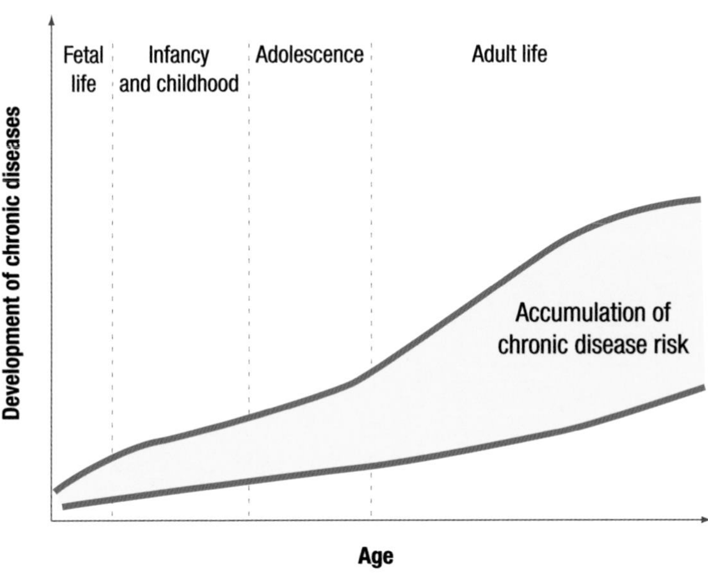

Source: reference *1*.

In general women live longer with chronic diseases than men, although they are in poor health (*271*). The costs associated with health care, including user fees, are a barrier to women's use of services. Women's income is lower than that of men, and they have less control over household resources. Chronic respiratory diseases require regular use of medicines. Therefore they are no exception to this rule.

In low and middle income countries, the exposure of women and children to biomass fuels is of great concern. Improving the health of women in developing countries is one of the key Millennium Development Goals (*272*).

Several features related to gender constitute specific risk factors for chronic respiratory diseases. For example, in many low income countries women are more exposed to the smoke of biomass fuels used for cooking, whereas in some other regions men are more often smokers. These explain some of the differences in the prevalence of asthma, allergic diseases and chronic obstructive pulmonary disease.

10. Tobacco Smoking: The Major Threat in High Income Countries, As Well As in Low And Middle Income Countries

KEY MESSAGES

- **Exposure to tobacco smoke, both the active and second hand, is a major threat to people in high income countries, as well as in low and middle income countries, because of its close link with noncommunicable and communicable diseases.**
- **The cumulative effect of tobacco smoke and other air pollutants increases the risk for chronic respiratory diseases.**

The spread of the tobacco epidemic is facilitated through a variety of complex factors with cross-border effects, including trade liberalization and direct foreign investment. Other factors such as global marketing, transnational tobacco advertising, promotion, lobbying and sponsorship, as well as international smuggling and counterfeit cigarettes, also contribute to the explosive increase in tobacco use.

Rates of tobacco use among 13–15 year old school children are high. The Global Tobacco Surveillance System collaborative group has recently analysed a sample of 747 603 adolescents from different countries and continents. They report the frequency of current tobacco use to vary from 11.4% in the Western Pacific Region, to 22.2% in the Americas, for a global average of 17.3%. While in general girls smoke less than boys, both in the Americas and in Europe, in the leading regions in smoking youngsters, the frequency is almost the same between genders (*273*).

Figure 18 The four stages of the tobacco epidemic

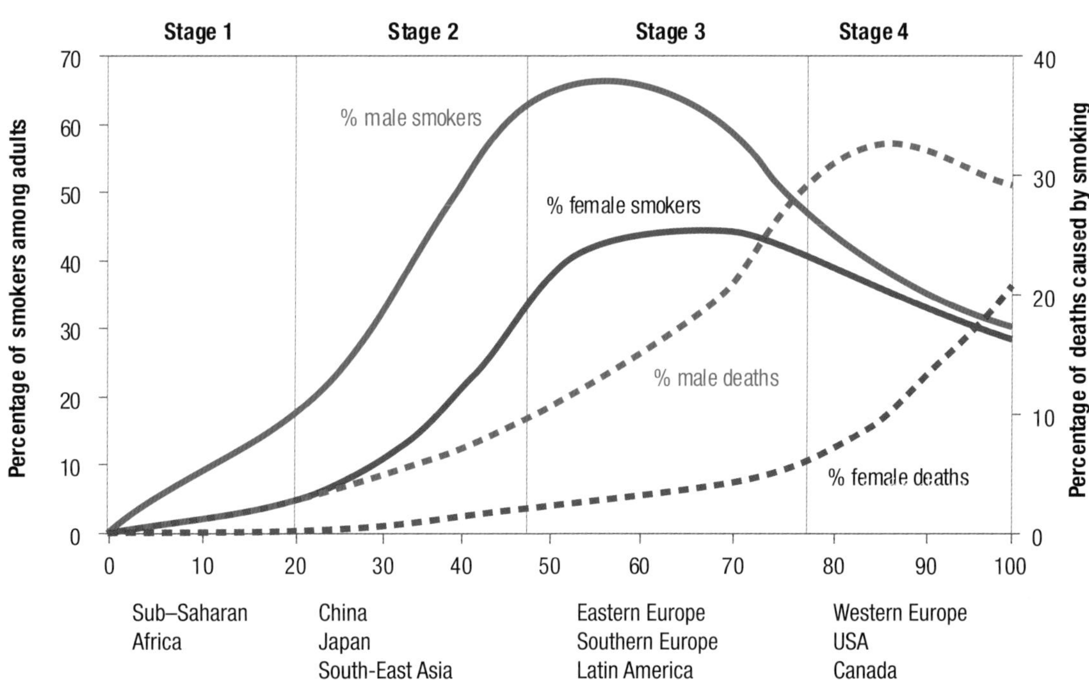

Source: reference *274* and *277*.

Smoking: the well-known killer

The report on *The Millennium Development Goals and tobacco control: an opportunity for global partnership* (*274*) summarizes the health effects of smoking. Tobacco is the second risk factor causing death after high blood pressure. The annual number of deaths from tobacco, estimated at nearly

Figure 19 Burden of disease attributable to selected environmental risk factors (percentage of DALYs in each subregion): (a) tobacco; (b) indoor smoke from solid fuels; (c) urban air pollution

(a) Tobacco

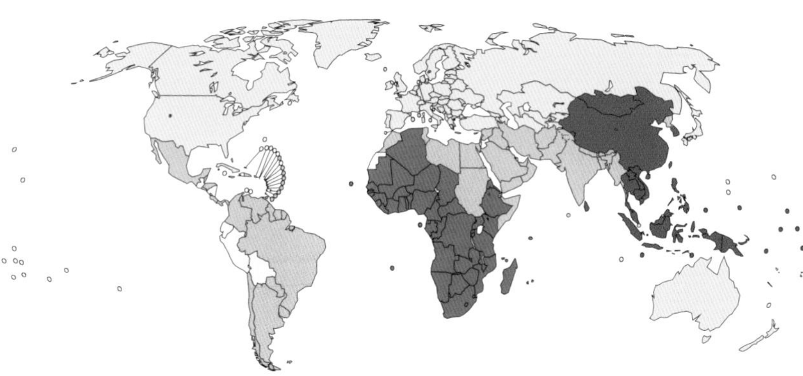

(b) Indoor smoke from solid fuels

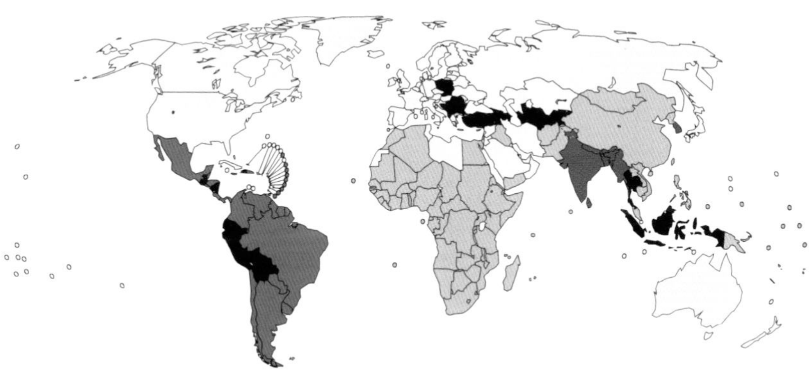

(c) Urban air pollution

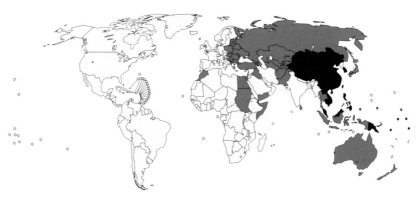

Proportion of DALYs attributable to selected risk factor

>0.5%	2–3.9%	16%+
0.5–0.9%	4–7.9%	
1–1.9%	8–15.9%	

Source: reference *7*.

5 million in 2000, was divided almost equally between high income and low and middle income countries (*275*). On current trends, mortality will increase to 8.3 million a year by 2030, and 80% of these deaths will occur in low and middle income countries (*276*) (Figures 18 and 19).

The leading causes of death from smoking are cardiovascular diseases (1.7 million deaths annually), chronic obstructive pulmonary disease (1 million deaths annually) and lung cancer (0.85 million deaths annually) (*275*). Patterns of death and disease from tobacco vary depending on the country's level of development (Figure 20).

Figure 20 Burden of disease attributable to tobacco and indoor smoke from solid fuel

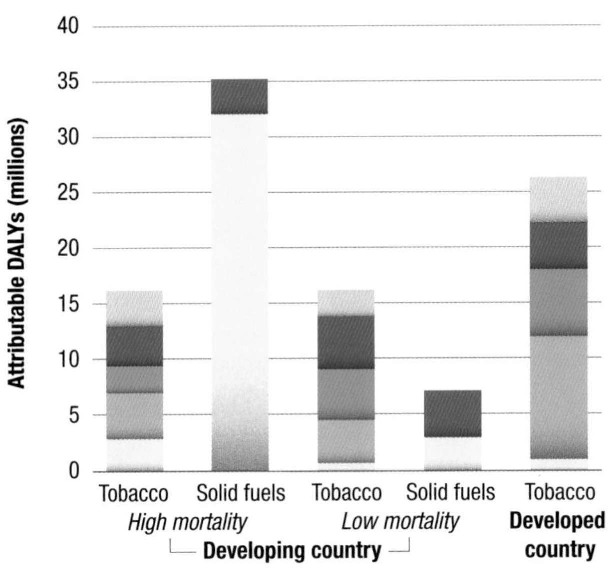

Source: reference *198*.

In the United States, vascular disease and lung cancer predominate. In China, chronic obstructive pulmonary disease causes more tobacco-related deaths than lung cancer. In India, with almost half the world's tuberculosis deaths, smoking exacerbates the effects of tuberculosis, and causes a greater risk of death. Tobacco is also responsible for a large portion of the disease burden in low and middle income countries and is the largest contributor to DALYs lost in high income countries (*278*).

Manufactured cigarettes, as well as all other products of "smoked tobacco" (e.g. cigars, or other "traditional" products like waterpipes, kreteks and bidis) are not the only form of tobacco that carries significant risk (*279*). All tobacco products are harmful and addictive and all can cause disease and death (*280, 281*).

Smokeless tobacco products (i.e. chewing tobacco, snuff, Swedish snus gutkha and other oral smokeless tobacco) used by many poor people – and especially by women – contain addictive levels of nicotine, many carcinogens, heavy metals, and other toxins and therefore carry a substantial mortality risk (*282*).

In low and middle income countries, tobacco smoking is linked with poverty and poor education (*283*). At the individual and household level, a lot of money is spent on tobacco. For poor people, money spent on tobacco is money not spent on basic necessities, such as food, shelter, education and health care. Tobacco users are at much higher risk of falling ill and dying prematurely of tobacco-related diseases, thus depriving families of much-needed income and imposing additional health-care costs. Those who grow tobacco suffer as well. Many tobacco farmers, rather than becoming rich from their crop, often find themselves in debt to tobacco companies (*283*).

Second-hand tobacco smoke

Second-hand tobacco smoke is the combination of smoke emitted from the burning end of a cigarette or other tobacco products and smoke exhaled by the smoker. Second-hand tobacco smoke contains thousands of known chemicals, at least 250 of which are known to be carcinogenic or otherwise toxic (*284*). Second-hand tobacco smoke is a major constituent of air pollution in indoor environments, including the home. Scientific evidence has firmly established that there is no safe level of exposure to second-hand tobacco smoke, a pollutant that causes serious illnesses in adults and children. In light of the accumulated evidence, local and national governments worldwide are increasingly implementing smoke-free policies in workplaces and public places to protect people from the dangers of second-hand tobacco smoke. Jurisdictions that have implemented smoke-free workplaces and public places have observed an immediate drop in levels of second-hand tobacco smoke, a decline in levels of second- hand tobacco smoke components in the population as well as significant and immediate health improvements in workers previously exposed to second-hand tobacco smoke.

In some countries, regulation on smoking in the workplace and public places has made the home the dominant unregulated source of environmental tobacco smoke. However, in most countries, the consequence of workplace exposure seems to be more serious than domestic exposure (*285*).Evidence on the adverse health effects of exposure to second-hand tobacco smoke has been accumulating for nearly 50 years. In children, environmental tobacco smoke increases the risk of sudden infant death syndrome, middle ear disease, lower respiratory tract illness, and prevalence of wheeze and cough. It also exacerbates asthma. In adults, environmental tobacco smoke is associated with an increased risk of chronic respiratory diseases, lung cancer and cancers of other sites (*286*), as well as cardiovascular disease (*287*). Intrauterine and environmental exposure to parental tobacco smoking is related to more respiratory symptoms and poorer lung function in adulthood.

There is no safe level of exposure to second-hand tobacco smoke (*284, 288–289*). Therefore, the elimination of smoking from indoor environments is the only science-based measure that adequately protects a population's health from the dangerous effects of second-hand tobacco smoke. Smoke-free policies protect health; where they are introduced, exposure to second-hand tobacco smoke falls and health improves. They are also extremely cost-effective, especially compared with the ineffective "alternatives" promoted by the tobacco industry, generally through third parties, namely (*284*):

- Separation of smokers and non-smokers within the same airspace.
- Increased ventilation and air filtration combined with "designated smoking areas."

11. Indoor Air Pollutants: The Unrecognized Killers In Low and Middle Income Countries

KEY MESSAGES

- **Solid fuels represent a major danger for health in low and middle income countries.**
- **Children under 5 years of age and women are the most vulnerable population because they are most likely to be exposed to indoor air pollution every day.**

Solid fuels represent a major danger in low and middle income countries. However, more than 3 billion people, almost all in low and middle income countries, rely on solid fuels, in the form of wood, dung and crop residues, for domestic energy (*272, 291, 292*). These materials are typically burnt in simple stoves with incomplete combustion. Consequently, women and young children are exposed to high levels of indoor air pollution every day resulting in an estimated 1.5–1.8 million premature deaths a year (*7, 270*). In Africa, approximately 1 million of these deaths occur in children aged under 5 years as a result of acute respiratory infections, 700 000 occur as a result of chronic obstructive pulmonary disease and 120 000 are attributable to cancer in adults, particularly in women (*292–301*). The global estimates may be up to 5 times higher. In a population survey in India, traditional solid fuels such as wood were found to have adverse effects on pulmonary function, in particular in women (*302*). It has been estimated, based on a model, that household indoor air pollution will cause a cumulative total of 9.8 million premature deaths by the year 2030 (*303*). In high income countries such as Spain, a strong association has been found between exposure to wood or charcoal smoke and chronic obstructive pulmonary disease (*304*), suggesting that the risks associated with the use of solid fuels may not be restricted to low and middle income countries.

Several indoor air pollutants are associated with asthma and chronic obstructive pulmonary disease (*292*). The main health pollutants in dwellings are second-hand tobacco smoke, indoor allergens, nitrogen oxide, formaldehyde, volatile organic compounds, indoor-generated particulate matter and carbon monoxide. These pollutants can affect the respiratory system and can cause or exacerbate asthma, acute respiratory diseases or chronic obstructive pulmonary disease. Some pollutants, such as radon, second-hand tobacco smoke and volatile organic compounds, pose a significant cancer risk. Among all indoor air pollutants, tobacco smoke is the major cause of indoor air pollution, morbidity and mortality in high, middle and low income countries (*305*).

12. Outdoor Air Pollutants

KEY MESSAGES

- **Urban air pollution poses a health risk worldwide, especially in low- and middle-income countries.**
- **Outdoor air pollutants have been associated with increased morbidity and mortality due to cardiovascular and respiratory diseases.**

Impact of air pollution on mortality and morbidity increases with the exposure levels but there are no thresholds below which the adverse effects of the pollution do not occur. Therefore the morbidity and mortality is increased by the pollution in all parts of the world, but at least half of the disease burden is borne by the populations of developing countries. People with existing heart or lung disease are at increased risk of acute symptoms or mortality (*306*).

Adverse respiratory health effects of air pollution are:

- Increased mortality.
- Increased incidence of cancer.
- Increased frequency of symptomatic asthma attacks.
- Increased incidence of lower respiratory infections.
- Increased exacerbations of disease in people with cardiopulmonary diseases, which could result in:
  - decreased ability to cope with daily activities (e.g. shortness of breath);
  - increased hospitalization, both in frequency and duration;
  - increased number of visits to emergency ward or physician;
  - increased need for pulmonary medication;
  - decreased pulmonary function.
- Reduction in FEV_1 or FVC associated with clinical symptoms:
  - in the short term (during acute exposure);
  - in the long term, marked by an increased rate of decline in pulmonary function.
- Increased prevalence of wheezing in the chest apart from colds, or of wheezing most days or nights.
- Increased prevalence or incidence of chest tightness.

- Increased prevalence or incidence of cough or phlegm production requiring medical attention.

- Increased incidence of acute upper respiratory infections that may interfere with normal activity.

- Eye, nose and throat irritation that may interfere with normal activity.

Long-term exposure to traffic-related air pollution may shorten life expectancy. Long-term exposure to combustion-related fine particulate air pollution is an important environmental risk factor for cardiac, pulmonary and lung cancer mortality (*307*). Even relatively low levels of air pollution observed in California, United States of America, have chronic, adverse effects on lung development in children from the age of 10 to 18 years, leading to clinically significant deficits in attained FEV_1 as children reach adulthood (*308, 309*).

The role of outdoor air pollution in causing chronic obstructive pulmonary disease or asthma needs to be studied further in order to separate out the effects of single pollutants from the combined effects of the complex mixture of air pollutants in urban atmospheres (*310*). The impact of outdoor air pollution appears to be smaller than that of cigarette smoke and indoor pollution (in respect of chronic obstructive pulmonary disease) and that of allergens (in respect of asthma) (*107, 311–314*). Outdoor air pollutants are of particular concern in low and middle income countries (*315*).

13. Allergens

KEY MESSAGES

- **Indoor and outdoor allergens are common in all countries.**
- **Exposure to allergens is one of the major triggers in sensitized individuals with asthma.**

Allergic diseases result from a complex interaction between genes, allergens (*316*) and co-factors which vary between regions (*317*). Allergens are antigens reacting with specific IgE antibodies. Allergens originate from a wide range of mites, animals, insects, plants, fungi or are small molecular weight chemicals. They are usually classified as indoor allergens (mites, some moulds, animal danders, insects) or outdoor allergens (pollens and some moulds). The role of allergens in the development of asthma is well established (*314*), although some uncertainties remain (*37*). Exposure to allergens is a trigger for symptoms in sensitized individuals with asthma. This is especially true for

Table 17 Prevalence of asthma and specific IgE in the 36 centres of the European Community Respiratory Health Survey (ECRHS I)

Countries[a]	Number of centres	Prevalence (%)		Odds ratio (95% CI)			
		Asthma	Atopy[b]	HDM[c]	Cat	Timothy grass	Atopy[b]
Estonia	1	7	18	1.82	8.74	3.12	1.25
Iceland	1	3	23	8.91	7.02	4.59	4.21
Spain	5	4–11	17–42	1.48–4.54	2.78–8.90	1.62–4.02	1.33–5.44
Norway	1	7	26	3.17	5.46	2.76	5.16
Italy	3	6–15	24–30	2.53–5.30	1.10–9.51	2.76–4.52	2.94–4.85
Sweden	3	8–10	30–32	1.88–2.36	2.60–5.54	2.02–3.58	1.92–5.17
France	4	6–13	29–43	1.79–4.64	3.43–6.48	1.37–3.98	1.53–4.60
Belgium	2	5–9	35–36	3.65–3.65	2.78–5.03	4.17–5.10	4.24–5.28
Germany	2	3–7	35–40	0.23–2.55	2.60–4.47	1.35–2.55	1.36–3.31
United Kingdom	4	9–14	34–44	2.01–5.07	2.33–5.17	1.62–2.86	2.03–5.74
Netherlands	3	5–7	36–41	2.06–6.14	3.75–5.52	2.44–5.49	2.03–5.74
Ireland	1	12	41	3.15	3.62	5.51	2.07
New Zealand	3	11–14	40–46	1.74–6.14	0.83–8.34	2.19–3.14	1.57–4.58
USA	1	12	43	1.01	2.13	2.48	2.52
Switzerland	1	10	45	1.86	1.31	1.75	1.53
Australia	1	12	45	2.89	3.24	2.41	3.22
All (95% CI)	36	9 (8–10)	34 (31–37)	2.78 (2.41–3.20)	4.18 (3.54–4.93)	2.63 (2.30–4.93)	2.82 (2.44–3.28)

[a] Countries listed in order of percentage of atopy.
[b] Atopy: any of house dust mite, cat, timothy grass, C. *herbarum*, and birch, Parietaria or ragweed IgE.
[c] House dust mite.
Source: reference *320*.

allergens primarily found indoors but can also be true for outdoor allergens with sufficiently high exposure (*319*) (Table 17).

Allergic sensitization is common in low and middle income countries, although some allergens may be specific to tropical environments (*321*). In Africa, allergic diseases are more common in urban than rural areas (*322, 323*), possibly because parasites protect people from atopic diseases (*324*). In deprived populations within the United States, cockroaches are common allergens (*325*).

14. Occupational Exposure

KEY MESSAGES

- **The workplace environment contributes significantly to the burden of chronic respiratory diseases.**
- **Because of the variation in latency periods, chronic respiratory diseases may occur immediately or only after many years.**

Workplace fatalities, injuries and illnesses remain at unacceptably high levels. They involve an enormous and unnecessary health burden, they cause great suffering, and they represent economic losses amounting to 4%–5% of GDP. According to ILO estimates for 2000, there are 2 million work-related deaths per year. WHO estimates that only 10%–15% of workers have access to a basic standard of occupational health services (*326*).

In 2000, WHO estimated that risk factors at the workplace were responsible worldwide for 37% of back pain, 16% of hearing loss, 13% of chronic obstructive pulmonary disease, 11% of asthma, 8% of injuries, 9% of lung cancer, and 2% of leukaemia. These risks at work caused 850 000 deaths worldwide and resulted in the loss of about 24 million years of healthy life (*327*).

Work-related respiratory conditions can have long latency periods. Once the disease process has begun, the worker continues to be at risk for many years, even after exposure ceases. In addition, once these conditions have developed, they are usually chronic and may worsen, even after avoidance of the risk factors.

Occupational respiratory diseases include a spectrum of conditions caused by the inhalation of both organic and inorganic materials (*328*). The population attributable risk of asthma and chronic obstructive pulmonary disease arising from work exposure is estimated to be up to 15% (*328*). Worldwide, asthma is the principal disease caused by the inhalation of organic agents. Fibrosis and cancers are the principal ailments resulting from inorganic agents: fibrosis in relation to silica dust (*329*) and asbestos, and fibrosis of the pleura and malignant mesothelioma in relation to asbestos fibers (*330–332*). Mesothelioma and lung cancers are now more frequent causes of death than asbestosis. Mortality attributable to asbestosis decreased over the last few decades of the 20th century because of the progressive implementation of workplace controls (*333*). Mesothelioma, in particular, is often related to a history of exposure to asbestos over a short period of time, often many years earlier. Smoking and tuberculosis are major co-factors in the development of occupational chronic respiratory diseases and cancers (*38, 334, 335*).

The workplace environment contributes significantly to the general burden of asthma (*336–338*) and COPD (*339*), but information on prevalence is difficult to obtain in many low and middle income countries. The worldwide mortality and morbidity from asthma, COPD, and pneumoconiosis arising from occupational airborne exposure were estimated for the year 2000 (*340*). There were an estimated 386 000 deaths (asthma, 38 000; COPD, 318 000; pneumoconiosis, 30 000) and nearly 6.6 million DALYs (asthma, 1 621 000; COPD, 3 733 000; pneumoconiosis, 1 288 000) attributable to exposure to occupational airborne particulates. Work-related asthma is the United Kingdom's fastest growing occupational disease and all health-care professionals should be aware of this possible diagnosis in patients with symptoms of asthma Patients with occupational asthma have higher rates of hospitalization and mortality than healthy workers (*341*).

In all countries, occupational chronic respiratory diseases represent a public health problem with economic implications (*13*). Technologies which are obsolete or banned in industrialized countries are still largely used in the world's poorest countries (*342*). In low and middle income countries, occupational illnesses are generally less visible and are not adequately recognized as a problem. Moreover, in those countries, most patients are not compensated and usually continue to work until the disease is severe and debilitating.

15. Diet and Nutrition

KEY MESSAGES

- **Dietary factors may be harmful or protective for chronic respiratory diseases.**
- **A dietary approach for the prevention and control of major chronic diseases could be beneficial for chronic respiratory diseases.**

For a long time, nutritional intake has been related to disease. WHO has adopted a broad-ranging approach under the Global Strategy on Diet, Physical Activity and Health, endorsed by the World Health Assembly in May 2004 (resolution WHA57.17). Dietary factors which increase or decrease the risk of other chronic diseases may be harmful or beneficial for chronic respiratory diseases (*343, 344*).

- Based on currently available evidence, it is not possible to conclude on the effect of dietary salt reduction in the management of asthma. However, there is an improvement in pulmonary function with a low salt diet. Further large-scale trials are required before any firm conclusions can be reached (*345*).

- Epidemiological studies suggest that a diet high in marine fatty acids (fish oil) may have beneficial effects on inflammatory conditions such as asthma (*346*). Fish oil supplementation has shown inconsistent effects in asthma outcomes (*347*).

- A beneficial effect of fresh fruit consumption on symptoms or lung function has been observed in asthma by several epidemiologic studies (*343, 348–350*). The role of vitamin C supplementation in the management of asthma is not clear yet (*351*).

- Obesity is a major risk factor of diabetes, cardiovascular diseases and other chronic diseases. It appears to be associated with the increased prevalence of asthma in high income (*16, 352–355*) and low and middle income countries as well as in deprived populations (*356*, *357*). Moreover, for people with asthma, obesity is a risk factor for dyspnea (*358*) and poor control of the disease (*359, 360*). Properly controlled studies are needed to confirm the benefits of weight-loss programmes for people with asthma (*361*). For people with COPD, obesity is thought to be a risk factor for dyspnea and may increase the severity of the disease (*201*).

  WHO dietary guidelines recommend exclusively breast-feeding for six month, in general. Studies suggest that exclusively breast-feeding, avoiding solid foods, seems to be effective for allergy prevention (*362*).

- A high proportion of COPD patients experience a significant weight loss, and low BMI is a marker of a poor prognosis (*363, 364*). Progressive weight loss in these patients is characterized by disease-specific elevated energy requirements that are unbalanced by dietary intake (*365*).

- Increases in the BMI of rural children in subsistence economies may lead to an increased prevalence of atopic disease (*366*).

Although diet and nutrition are not major direct risk factors for chronic respiratory diseases, obesity can be associated with dyspnoea and further increment the symptoms of chronic respiratory diseases.

16. Post-infectious Chronic Respiratory Diseases

Respiratory infections are common in low and middle income countries, but their consequences of are not often reported (*367*) and no true prevalence can be obtained since there is a lack of accurate data. Bronchiectasis is common after viral infections in children (*368*). Severe sequelae resulting from tuberculosis include bronchiectasis, pachypleuritis, aspergillosis or fibrothorax (*369–371*). It seems that a high proportion of tuberculosis deaths are attributable to post-tuberculosis chronic respiratory disease, but data are lacking to support this assertion. In high income countries also, respiratory tract infections in children and adolescents can cause chronic respiratory diseases in adult life (*372*). The interactions with smoking or HIV/AIDS have a major deleterious effect.

There is now extensive evidence from many countries that conditions before birth and in early childhood influence health in adult life (*373*). Children are unable to choose the environment in which they live, their diet, living situation, and exposure to tobacco smoke and other air pollutants. They also have a very limited ability to understand the long-term consequences of their behaviour. Yet it is precisely during this crucial phase that many health behaviours are shaped. Young tobacco smokers, for example, may acquire the habit and become dependent well before reaching adulthood.

STEPWISE FRAMEWORK FOR ACTION

17. GARD Approach

KEY MESSAGES

- **GARD will work at international and national level.**
- **GARD's planning steps correspond to WHO's strategic objectives and action plans.**
- **GARD will exploit synergies, building on and complementing existing programmes and projects.**

The Global Alliance against Chronic Respiratory Diseases (GARD) is a voluntary alliance of national and international organizations, institutions and agencies working towards the common goal of improving global lung health. The Alliance is part of WHO's global work to prevent and control chronic diseases, based on the stepwise framework (Figure 21) set out in *Preventing chronic diseases: a vital investment* (*1*).

Figure 21 Stepwise framework

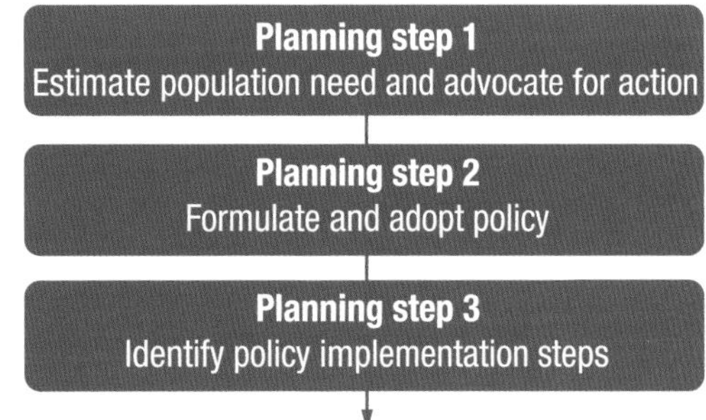

Policy implementation steps	Population–wide interventions National level	 Sub-national level	Interventions for individuals
Implementation step 1 **Core**	Interventions that are feasible to implement with existing resources in the short term		
Implementation step 2 **Expanded**	Interventions that are feasible to implement with a realistic projected increase in or reallocation of resources in the medium term		
Implementation step 3 **Desirable**	Evidence-based interventions beyond the reach of existing resources		

Source: reference *1*.

Planning step 1: estimate population need and advocate for action

The basis for action is to estimate disease burden and population needs, identify risk factors for chronic respiratory diseases and respiratory allergies, and undertake surveillance on chronic respiratory disease risk factors, and trends in disease burden, as well as in costs, quality and affordability of care. The data will need to be compared between countries (high–income, and low- and middle-income) to define strategies for policy-makers and to assess the impact of chronic respiratory diseases programmes. There is also a need to advocate for action to combat chronic respiratory diseases in order to raise awareness among all stakeholders and make chronic respiratory diseases a public health priority in all countries.

With this in mind, GARD will assess needs and objectives, and propose a plan of action for future GARD activities.

Planning step 2: formulate and adopt policy

In all countries, a national policy and planning framework is essential to allocate chronic diseases appropriate priority and to ensure that resources are organized efficiently (*11*). GARD will provide the basis for action in the field of chronic respiratory diseases, with plans for the implementation of policies. Implementation will start with pilot studies, developed by local experts and stakeholders in each country, relevant to the needs, resources and setting of that country.

Comprehensive and integrated policies and plans for prevention are vital because they minimize overlap and fragmentation in the health system. Policies and plans to prevent chronic respiratory diseases should therefore (*1, 11*):

- Cut across specific diseases and focus on common risk factors' since many risk factors, such as tobacco smoking and other air pollutants, affect many different diseases.
- Encompass promotion, prevention and control strategies.
- Emphasize a population-based approach, rather than targeting specific subgroups.
- Integrate activities across settings, such as health-care centres, schools, workplaces and communities.
- Link with other government programmes and community-based actions.

Risk factors induce different diseases (Table 18), and some risk factors should only be targeted in some areas.

Many low-income countries may find it difficult to draw up control strategies for specific chronic diseases. They may opt to use integrated programmes already developed by WHO, covering communicable and chronic respiratory diseases for example, the Practical Approach to Lung Health (PAL) (*374–376*)

Table 18 Diseases resulting from exposure to risk factors

	Chronic respiratory diseases	Cardiovascular diseases	Respiratory cancer	Others major diseases
Active and second-hand smoking	+	+	+	Other cancers, diabetes
Solid fuels, indoors	+		+	Acute respiratory infections
Other indoor air pollutants	+	+	+	
Outdoor air pollutants	+	+	+	
Allergens	+			Allergic diseases
Inhaled occupational agents	+		+	
Diet and nutrition	±	+	+	Diabetes
Post-infection	+			

and the Practical Approach to Lung Health in South Africa (PALSA Plus) (*22*). In middle-income countries, however, some disease-specific plans already exist, for example the asthma plan in China, and the asthma and rhinitis plan in Brazil (Table 19). GARD therefore proposes a strategy which combines a syndromic approach (PAL and PALSA Plus) with a disease-specific approach (focusing on asthma and rhinitis, COPD, occupational chronic respiratory disease, and pulmonary hypertension). Since many countries will not have sufficient resources currently available to implement the entire policy, countries will need to decide on the best plan according to their priorities, resources, health systems and intersectoral possibilities.

Table 19 Some examples of countries with a national plan on chronic respiratory diseases

Country	Plan	Comments
Brazil	Asthma and rhinitis	in primary health care
China	Asthma, COPD	surveillance and awareness
Finland	Asthma, COPD	broad long term intervention
France	Asthma, COPD	
Portugal	Asthma, COPD	
USA	Asthma	

In the future, a syndromic approach will be developed for middle- and high-income countries (GARD implementation steps 2 and 3).

A policy or plan on chronic respiratory diseases should:

- **Promote health through the prevention of chronic respiratory diseases and respiratory allergies:** by reducing the burden of tobacco smoke and other types of indoor and outdoor pollution, occupational hazards and other relevant risk factors.

- **Recommend simple and affordable diagnostic tools for the diagnosis of chronic respiratory diseases and respiratory allergies:** taking account of the different health needs, the services to be provided and the resources available, as well as the need for adequate training of health professionals in the use of the tools.

- **Control chronic respiratory diseases and allergies, and ensure drug accessibility:**

    - in areas with a high burden of communicable diseases and a functioning primary health care service, by promoting models such as PAL;

    - in areas with a high prevalence of HIV infection, by promoting models such as PALSA Plus;

    - by using different models of prevention and care for chronic respiratory diseases in middle- and high-income countries to target asthma, rhinitis, chronic obstructive pulmonary diseases and occupational lung diseases;

    - by ensuring a focus on the control of occupational chronic respiratory diseases, sleep apnea syndrome and pulmonary hypertension, which have been insufficiently considered worldwide.

The key aspects of GARD action plans at national level will be:

- to ensure the availability of drugs in each treatment setting for patients with chronic respiratory diseases;

- to assist in the training of health-care workers in the management of chronic respiratory diseases to ensure that they are able to identify feasible options and then set priorities on the basis of current evidence;

- Develop a specific action plan for paediatric chronic respiratory diseases and respiratory allergies: covering chronic respiratory diseases in childhood and adolescence.

Planning step 3: identify policy implementation steps

Health priorities, geographic variability in risk factors and chronic respiratory diseases, the diversity of national health-care service systems and variations in the availability and affordability of treatments, all require that any recommendations should be adapted locally to ensure their appropriateness to the community in which they will be applied. GARD action plans developed during the planning step 2 will be collated and rolled out to as many countries as possible. The policy implementation process will follow the stepwise framework (*1*), and the results will be measurable:

- **Implementation step 1 (core):** interventions that are feasible to implement with existing resources in the short term.

- **Implementation step 2 (expanded):** interventions that are possible to implement with a realistically projected increase in, or reallocation of, resources in the medium term.

- **Implementation step 3 (desirable):** evidence-based interventions that are beyond the reach of existing resources.

The following chapters outline GARD's role in support of the three planning steps:

- estimate population need and advocate for action (Chapters 18 and 19);

- formulate and adopt policy (Chapters 20–23);

- identify policy implementation steps (Chapter 24).

18. Estimate Burden, Identify Risk Factors and Undertake Surveillance

KEY MESSAGES

- **In all countries, the prevalence and incidence of chronic respiratory diseases are under-investigated.**
- **Epidemiological studies, with questionnaires and simple spirometry, are needed to properly estimate the burden of chronic respiratory diseases.**
- **Existing WHO databases should be integrated with the data on chronic respiratory disease morbidity rates and any other risk factor data.**

Basic epidemiological data on the chronic respiratory disease risk factors, burden and surveillance are reported for less than 25% of the world's population and are largely from high-income countries. However, it is the low- and middle-income countries which will experience the largest increase in chronic diseases (*372*). Data on chronic respiratory disease risk factors, burden and surveillance are fragmented and often incomplete in high-income countries. Prevalence and morbidity data can underestimate the burden of chronic respiratory diseases because these diseases are not usually diagnosed until they are clinically apparent and moderately advanced.

These failures make it difficult to raise awareness and to elaborate policies for the prevention, diagnosis and control of chronic respiratory diseases, and to predict future diseases in the population. Standard disease definitions and methods to monitor the burden and provide surveillance over time need to be improved.

What will GARD do?

GARD will develop a standardized process to obtain data on chronic respiratory disease risk factors, trends in disease burden, and quality and affordability of care, as well as the economic burden. These data can then be compared between countries (high- middle– and low-income) in order to identify strategies for policy-makers and to assess the impact of chronic respiratory disease programmes.

Based on both WHO and non-WHO activities (Box 4), GARD will create an inventory of studies that have collected data on:

- The prevalence and severity of diseases, as well as their risk factors.
- The social and economic burden of chronic respiratory diseases.

GARD will also:

- Support countries in obtaining baseline measures and in monitoring trends in the burden of chronic respiratory diseases.
- Expand WHO internal initiatives in countries (such as the stepwise approach to surveillance (WHO-STEPS) and the Global InfoBase programmes).

With regard to the stepwise approach to surveillance of chronic respiratory diseases, GARD proposes the following activities (Figure 22):

Step 1. Collect questionnaire-based information on tobacco use and any other indoor and outdoor pollution and respiratory symptoms. For asthma, the International Study of Asthma and Allergy in Childhood (ISAAC) and the European Community Respiratory Health Survey (ECRHS) questionnaires are available (*378, 379*). For COPD, several questionnaires, including the Burden of Chronic Obstructive Lung Disease (BOLD) questionnaire, are available (*164, 380, 381*).

Step 2. Use standardized physical examination and spirometry. Ideally, low-cost spirometry should be available in primary health care centres.

Step 3. Expand testing to full lung-function tests, oxymetry and allergy tests.

Figure 22 GARD proposal for the stepwise approach to surveillance of chronic respiratory diseases

SURVEILLANCE OF MAJOR CHRONIC RESPIRATORY DISEASES ACCORDING TO WHO-STEPS (1)

Step 1: Questionnaire–based assessment

Step 2: + Physical assessment Simple objective measures (e.g. peak flow meter)

Step 3: + more expensive or time consuming tests (e.g. methacholine challenge, skin prick test, IgE testing, reversibility test, blood gas measurement, alpha–1–antitrypsin)

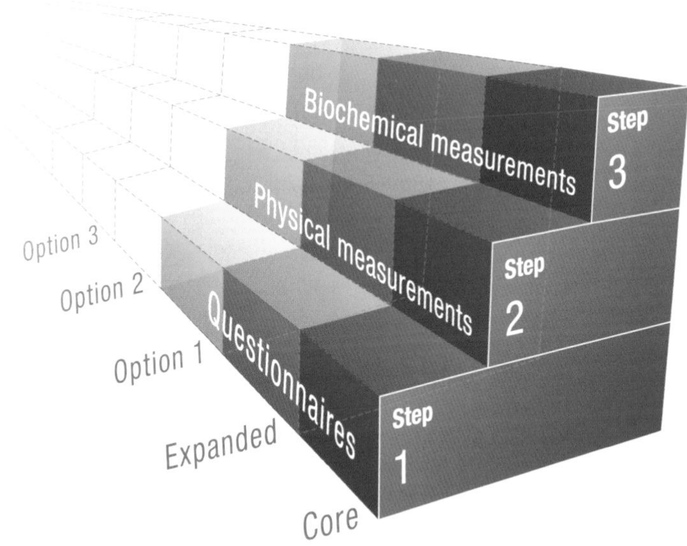

Box 4 Surveillance: sources of information

Estimates of burden and mortality attributable to chronic respiratory diseases are needed to support advocacy. Information on which to base such estimates is available from a variety of sources, as listed below.

WHO sources

The WHO stepwise approach to surveillance (WHO-STEPS) is a standardized tool to help low- and middle-income countries assess the risk factors of chronic diseases, (www.who.int/ncd_surveillance/infobase). WHO-STEPS focuses on building capacity in low- and middle-income countries in order to collect small amounts of high-quality data on risk factors.

WHO surveillance of risk factors (SuRF) displays data on prevalence and mean values of eight major risk factors related to chronic diseases, for WHO Member States (www.who.int/ncd_surveillance/infobase). SuRF responds to the fundamental need of public health systems to invest in surveillance.

CONTINUED ON NEXT PAGE

BOX 4 (CONTINUED)

WHO questionnaire for national surveys of chronic respiratory disease capacity is a standardized and validated questionnaire that can be used to assess the national capacity for surveillance, prevention, and control of chronic respiratory diseases (*383*). It covers:

- Health indicators.
- Policies and operational plans.
- Legislation.
- Information systems and statistics.
- Structure and financing of prevention and treatment activities.
- Availability of national guidelines.
- Nature of available services.
- Human resources.
- Role of nongovernmental organizations.
- Capacity for monitoring and evaluation.
- Drug availability.

WHO study on prevalence of major respiratory diseases at primary health care level in low- and middle-income countries is investigating:

- Prevalence and severity of respiratory diseases.
- Under-diagnosis and management of respiratory diseases.

A two-stage survey is envisaged. The first stage will be a survey of individuals, aged 6 years or over, attending a primary health care clinic. It consists of a brief questionnaire administered by a doctor or nurse or technician to obtain information on demographics, exposure to risk factors (primarily smoking, occupational and domestic exposure to particulates from using solid fuels, and migration), respiratory symptoms, diagnoses and comorbidities. At the same time, similar data will be collected from outpatients attending emergency room departments. The second stage will be a clinical survey of respiratory patients of the same age within the same setting attending primary health care clinics. A general practitioner will examine the patient and fill in a questionnaire about the diagnosis. After that, a measurement of lung function will be performed by a technician or nurse to estimate the "true" prevalence of airway obstruction at the primary health care level. Some of the patients will be selected by WHO experts to be later evaluated by a research team in order to validate the general practitioner's diagnosis. The respiratory patients will also complete the questionnaire used in the first stage. The respiratory diseases covered include asthma, COPD, tuberculosis, pneumonia and allergic rhinitis.

Other sources

Various international and national surveys have been conducted and published in recent years, providing the basis for current estimates of burden and mortality attributable to chronic respiratory diseases. The information they present, however, is represents only high- and middle-income countries. Such sources include:

- Burden of Chronic Obstructive Lung Disease (BOLD) (www.kpchr.org/public/studies/stds) (*164*).
- United States Department of Health and Human Services: *Healthy people 2010 goals for respiratory diseases* (http://hin.nhlbi.nih.gov/as_frameset.htm).

CONTINUED ON NEXT PAGE

BOX 4 (CONTINUED)

- **European Community Respiratory Health Survey (ECRHS) (www.ecrhs.org) (*378*).**
- **European Respiratory Society (ERS): *White book* (www.ersnet.org) (*125*).**
- **Global Initiative for Asthma (GINA): report on the burden of asthma (*15*).**
- **Indicators for monitoring COPD and asthma in the EU (IMCA) (europa.eu.int/comm/health/ph_projects/2001/monitoring).**
- **International Study of Asthma and Allergy in Childhood (ISAAC) (http://isaac.auckland.ac.nz) (*384*).**
- **United States National Heart, Lung, and Blood Institute (NHLBI): *Fact book 2003* (http://www.nhlbi.nih.gov/about/factpdf.htm) and *Chart book 2003* (http://www.nhlbi.nih.gov/resources/docs/cht-book.htm).**

Deliverables to be produced by GARD

To assist in estimating the burden of chronic respiratory diseases, identifying risk factors and carrying out surveillance, GARD will undertake the following activities:

- Comparison and evaluation of the strengths and weaknesses of existing programmes assessing the chronic respiratory disease burden and risk factors, with a focus on low- and middle-income countries.
- Elaboration and publication of two chronic respiratory disease modules to be incorporated in WHO-STEPS and the WHO Global InfoBase.
- Publication of an expanded and upgraded version of the existing WHO questionnaire used to assess and monitor the national chronic respiratory disease capacity.

19. Advocate for Action

KEY MESSAGES

- **Although the cost of inaction is clear and unacceptable, preventable chronic respiratory diseases and their risk factors receive insufficient attention from the health-care community, government officials, the media, patients and their families.**
- **Chronic respiratory diseases need to be higher up the health agenda of key policy-makers.**
- **All stakeholders should be involved in increasing awareness of chronic respiratory diseases.**
- **An important part of advocacy is to disseminate information, the ultimate goal of which is to provide evidence that the burden of chronic respiratory diseases can be reduced.**

Having set out a framework for the prevention and control of chronic respiratory diseases, it is essential to seek early commitment from potential partners. Advocacy helps to set the record straight and to spur action at all levels.

- Hundreds of millions of people are affected by preventable chronic respiratory diseases. Currently 300 million people have asthma, 210 million people have moderate to severe chronic obstructive pulmonary disease, while millions of others suffer from mild chronic obstructive pulmonary disease, allergic rhinitis and other often-undiagnosed chronic respiratory diseases (*30-32*).

- Preventable chronic respiratory diseases have major adverse effects on the quality of life and ability of affected individuals. They cause premature deaths and jeopardize the economic prospects of families, communities and societies in general.

- The huge burden attributable to chronic respiratory diseases is largely unknown because these diseases are not accorded priority on the public health agenda of any country.

- Lack of awareness results in lack of attention being paid to chronic respiratory diseases, in particular as regards prevention, early diagnosis and control. In most low- and middle-income countries, lack of financial support is a barrier to capacity development for prevention, treatment and research.

- Chronic respiratory diseases need to be higher up on the health agenda of key policy-makers. Advocacy is needed to provide policy-makers with convincing evidence about the possibility of controlling risk factors, and persuading them to set in motion health system changes necessary to do so.

What will GARD do?

In order to address effectively the global public health problems caused by chronic respiratory diseases, GARD will endeavour:

- To make chronic respiratory diseases a public health priority in all countries.

- To ensure that governments, the media, the public, patients and health-care professionals (including those in schools and workplaces) are aware of the magnitude of this problem and that, where needed, appropriate information on known effective interventions is disseminated.

GARD will therefore be dealing with both awareness and dissemination. The goal of awareness is to draw attention to the problem of chronic respiratory diseases, while that of dissemination is to provide information about what can specifically be done, or what is recommended.

Awareness

Despite growing evidence of epidemiological and economic impact, the global response to the problem of chronic diseases remains inadequate (*385*). The most important barrier to changing this unsatisfactory situation is the refusal to recognize the problem. There are 193 countries with different needs, priorities, economic status, health-care systems and it is impossible to convey a single message. A message about spirometry is not relevant to all of these countries because most cannot provide access to it for their populations.

In raising awareness, GARD will invite a broad range of stakeholders to contribute, including:

- **Governments.** The governments of countries where an action plan has been initiated have a critical role to play.

  - governments are concerned with the well-being of their citizens, and need to address the socioeconomic consequences of poor health status of the population. If governments show interest in health issues, then the media and the public will also be interested;

  - it is important that a high-level government official, such as the Minister of Health, acts as the spokesperson for the issue.

- **Physicians and other health-care professionals.** The medical community is an important target of an awareness campaign. While physicians know about chronic respiratory diseases, they are usually unaware of the effectiveness of prevention and management methods. Thus there is a need to disseminate information on appropriate and effective interventions for prevention and treatment.

- **Patients and the public at large.** GARD can reach patients and the general public through the media and the Internet. Newsworthy stories can be used to draw attention to chronic respiratory diseases. People are more aware of asthma because many famous athletes have competed on the world stage despite having asthma. COPD has not benefited in the same way, partly because of the stigma attached to patients because their diseases are regarded as their own fault.

- **The media.** The media represent a very potent vehicle in increasing public awareness, but the interest of the media is unlikely to be mobilized unless governments focus on the problem. With greater public awareness, patients and their families will in turn become more proactive about the conditions which affect them.

- **Private sector.** The pharmaceutical industry and manufacturers of diagnostic tools could be mobilized to play a role in raising awareness, subject to the strict rules applicable to private sector interaction with GARD (*27*).

- **Academic research groups.** One of the challenges of GARD will be to evaluate cost-effectiveness of various strategies for prevention and control of chronic respiratory diseases. This task can only be accomplished with the collaboration of academic research groups.

- **Nongovernmental organizations and foundations.** Nongovernmental organizations and foundations may provide invaluable brain power and financial resources.

- **United Nations agencies.** Aiming at health promotion and disease prevention, United Nations agencies could be of great help.

Box 5 The World Health Organization

WHO has the experience to implement awareness campaigns through local/country/regional governments and the commitment of WHO to support GARD is essential in ensuring its success. There are success stories and they must be communicated (albeit carefully) to officials of governments where GARD is implemented. One of these, Health and Environment Linkage Initiatives (HELI, www.who.int/heli/en/) is a global effort by WHO and UNEP (United Nations Environment Programme) to support action by low and middle income country policymakers on environmental threats to health. HELI encourages countries to address health and environment linkages as being integral to its economic development.

The World Health Assembly will not address GARD in the current year, but could do so in future years. The *WHO Bulletin* is also an effective tool.

An approach to reach all the target audiences is to add information about GARD to the ongoing relevant World Day Campaigns – World Asthma Day, World Allergy Day, and World COPD Day. All of these World Day Campaigns have been active for a number of years, and have reached a wide target audience in many countries. Each year, they have a theme, with activities conducted in a variety of settings. The public responds, as they have an interest in a specific disease, or a member of their family has that disease.

GARD could provide information (flyers, posters, documents) to be added to the materials for these ongoing World Day Campaigns. In preparing publicity materials, GARD should examine how awareness campaigns about other chronic diseases have been conducted (for example, hypertension, kidney diseases and diabetes). Perhaps, in due course, it might be appropriate to consider a specific GARD World Day.

Dissemination

GARD will also be involved with dissemination. Dissemination differs from awareness with regard to both target audience and content. The ultimate goal of dissemination of information about chronic respiratory diseases is to provide evidence that something can be done. Chronic respiratory diseases can be prevented using a variety of strategies and interventions. In addition, most patients with chronic respiratory diseases can be effectively treated. Governments, the public, and patients and their families need to receive these messages. In the absence of a positive message, no interest will develop and no changes will occur.

Health-care professionals are the main target of dissemination efforts concerning chronic respiratory diseases, albeit not the only one. Unfortunately, in many countries, medical education does not focus enough on chronic respiratory diseases and thus physicians and other health-care professionals may not be fully aware of what can be done. The Practical Approach to Lung Health (PAL) is a model that has worked. GARD should consider developing a global or regional educational programme about chronic respiratory diseases aimed at the medical profession. To do so, GARD should consider building partnerships with local or international professional societies.

20. Implement Prevention and Health Promotion

KEY MESSAGES

- **Everyone has the right to live and work in an environment where the air is clean.**
- **Environmental exposure to an unhealthy environment can cause severe and debilitating COPD, asthma, cardiovascular disease and cancer.**
- **Complete elimination of the risk factor is the only way to remove the risk, be it cigarette smoke, indoor or outdoor air pollution, allergens or occupational exposure.**

Health promotion is the process of enabling people to increase control over their health and its determinants. It is a core function of public health and a cornerstone of primary health care (*386*). The cost–effectiveness of any health-promotion programme should be carefully evaluated before the programme is implemented.

Health promotion and prevention programmes should focus on the major risk factors for chronic respiratory diseases. Smoking, solid fuel and occupational exposure are the most important ones, but other risk factors such as allergen exposure and outdoor pollution should also be considered. Long-term effects from the abatement of tobacco smoke, environmental exposure to tobacco smoke and outdoor air pollution are raising great expectations (*387*). Population-based strategies that seek to shift the distribution of risk factors often have the potential to produce substantial reductions in disease burden (*388*).

There are three levels of prevention (*389*):

- **Primary prevention** is the protection of health by personal and community-wide actions, e.g. preserving good nutritional status, physical activity and emotional well-being, immunizing against infectious diseases and making the environment safe.
- **Secondary prevention** encompasses the measures available to individuals and populations for early detection of departures from good health, and prompt and effective intervention to correct them.
- **Tertiary prevention** consists of the measures available to reduce or eliminate long-term impairments and disabilities, to minimize suffering caused by existing departures from good health, and to promote the patient's adjustment to irremediable conditions. This extends the concept of prevention to the field of rehabilitation (*390*). This chapter highlights some key points of disease prevention.

The chronic respiratory disease epidemic is in large part linked to risk factors. Many risk factors predisposing people to chronic respiratory diseases are preventable, but policy and legislation are still inadequate throughout the world, particularly in low– and middle–income countries. The Framework Convention on Tobacco Control (FCTC) is an international treaty that has been ratified by over 140 countries, but it has yet to been ratified by many other countries. Indoor pollution is a major cause of chronic respiratory diseases, especially in low– and middle–income countries. Many people, however, are still unaware of the damage to respiratory health caused by indoor pollutants. In many countries, harmful occupational exposure is a major cause of chronic respiratory diseases but workers are not protected adequately. Screening programmes and prevention in schools are the exception rather than the rule.

Countries should implement policies to reduce the burden of tobacco smoke, indoor and outdoor pollution, occupational hazards and other risk factors of relevance for chronic respiratory diseases. In support of such action, and in response to requests from countries, GARD will:

- Provide guidance on establishing programmes to prevent chronic respiratory diseases.

- Help countries to formulate national objectives and realistic timetables for their achievement.

- Develop a measurable process and output indicators for accurate monitoring and evaluation of actions.

In providing support to countries, GARD will seek synergies with existing activities (Box 6) in order to maximize the effect of its work.

What will GARD do?

GARD will work towards reducing exposure to the major risk factors for chronic respiratory diseases. To do so, GARD will promote – and support countries in implementing – the following important policies.

Ban smoking

Several countries and hundreds of local jurisdictions in the world have successfully implemented laws requiring indoor workplaces and public places to be 100% smoke-free without encountering significant challenges in enforcement. The evidence from these jurisdictions consistently demonstrates not only that smoke-free environments are enforceable, but that they are popular and become more so following implementation. These laws have no negative impact and often have a positive one, on businesses in the hospitality sector and elsewhere. Their outcomes, a likely reduction in heart attacks and respiratory problems, also have a positive impact on health. Developed and developing countries like Ireland, New Zealand, Scotland and Uruguay, have built on the implementation of smoke-free laws at the local level that began in North America in the late 1970s. With almost universal success, they have since enacted and implemented laws to protect workers and the public from second-hand smoke in almost all indoor workplaces and public places (including bars and casinos), achieving strong popular support. Other countries are interested in learning from their experiences.

Smoke-free workplaces result in lower levels of tobacco consumption among smokers and are associated with a greater likelihood of workers implementing smoke-free policies in their homes (*391-393*). Therefore, smoke-free workplace legislation should be a primary strategy in protecting individuals from second-hand smoke in their home. According to WHO Policy recommendations on protection from exposure to second-hand tobacco smoke (*394*), removing the pollutant —tobacco smoke — through implementation of 100% smoke-free environments is the only effective strategy to reduce exposure to tobacco smoke in indoor environments to safe levels and to provide an acceptable level of protection from the dangers of second-hand smoke exposure. Therefore, legislation that includes ventilation and smoking areas, whether separately ventilated from non-smoking areas or not, is not recommended.

GARD will promote legislation to ensure that:

- All workers can work in a smoke-free environment.
- Citizens can enjoy smoke-free public places.
- People who buy or rent a new house have smoke-free cooking options.

In order to prepare for a ban on smoking, GARD will:

- Encourage active role of legislators.
- Conduct campaigns to educate the general public, and patients and their families on the benefits of a smoke free indoor environment.
- Identify natural allies in the mainstream, such as trade unions and employers associations.
- Identify a number of independent "champions", including selected politicians.
- Track public opinion continuously and regularly publicize support.

The objective is to create (over a 3–year period) a favourable climate for legislation.

In terms of implementation, GARD will:

- Build enforcement mechanisms to ensure compliance when imposing a ban on smoking.
- Prevent introducing the smoking ban overnight, and support it only when enforcement mechanisms are ready.
- Establish confidential channels for complaints about violations of the smoking ban, so that inspections can focus on suspected cases of non-compliance.
- Make bar owners liable to fines and loss of license if they fail to implement the smoking ban.

- Conduct inspections in the months following the introduction of the smoking ban (in Ireland, 35 000 inspections were carried out in the first 9 months after the smoking ban was introduced, for an Irish population of 4 million).

- Publish success stories to create a landslide effect.

The indicator to be used to evaluate GARD's activity will be the number of countries that have benefited from GARD's support where a smoking ban has been approved and implemented according to the above terms.

Box 6 Prevention and promotion: potential synergies

WHO programmes on Health Promotion and Prevention

Numerous initiatives have contributed to health promotion and prevention of chronic respiratory diseases. Some are directly related to WHO, or are WHO activities, others are not. GARD should be able to help countries to formulate and adopt integrated policies in the field of chronic respiratory diseases.

WHO activities

- **WHO Framework Convention on Tobacco Control (WHO FCTC). This is the first international public health treaty, that reaffirms the right of all people to the highest standard of health. The WHO FCTC was initiated and negotiated under the auspices of the WHO (*393*)(www.who.int/tobacco). It was developed in response to the globalization of the tobacco epidemic (*392*). Since its entry into force on 27 February 2005, the Convention has attracted a high number of parties and has become one of the most widely embraced treaties in the history of the United Nations. Among its many measures, the treaty requires countries to impose restrictions on tobacco advertising, sponsorship and promotion; establish new packaging and labelling of tobacco products; establish clean indoor air controls; and strengthen legislation to clamp down on tobacco smuggling (e.g. increasing the tax and prices on tobacco products).**

- **Prevention of Allergy and Allergic Asthma. WHO has organized consultations and published publications in this field, addressing primary and secondary prevention (*396, 397, 398*).**

- **Programme on indoor air pollution (www.who.int/indoorair). WHO's programme on indoor air pollution focuses on:**

  - research and evaluation;
  - capacity building;
  - evidence for policy-makers.

- **Programme on Air Quality and Health (www.euro.who.int/air). The programme on Air Quality and Health programme of WHO based in Bonn, evaluates health risks of air pollutants producing WHO Air Quality Guidelines, supporting assessment of health risks of the pollution as well as development of tools helping in risk reduction.**

- **Programme on occupational chronic respiratory diseases. WHO addresses occupational health through a programme at WHO headquarters, in the six WHO regional offices and in WHO country offices, with the support of a network of 64 Collaborating Centres (www.who.int/occupational_health). WHO is implementing a global strategy to:**

  - provide evidence for policy, legislation and support to decision-makers, including work carried out to estimate the magnitude of the burden of occupational diseases and injuries;

BOX 6 (CONTINUED)

- provide infrastructure support and development through capacity building, information dissemination and networking;
- support protection and promotion of workers' health.

Other activities

- **European Environment and Health Committee.** The European Environment and Health Committee is a coalition that brings together representatives from health ministries, environment ministries, intergovernmental organizations and civil-society organizations. Its overall role is to support countries as they try to reduce environmental hazards that affect human health. It oversees coordination and follow-up of the outcomes of the environment and health process in the European Region, and helps to promote and ensure reporting back on the implementation of the commitments made at the Fourth Ministerial Conference on Environment and Health which took place in Budapest in June 2004. The WHO Regional Office for Europe is a member of European Environment and Health Committee (www.euro.who.int).
- **Children's Environment and Health Action Plan for Europe.** The Children's Environment and Health Action Plan for Europe was launched in 1989 with the aim of eliminating the most significant environmental threats to health as rapidly as possible. It takes the approach that prevention is better than cure. Progress is marked by a ministerial conferences, held every five years. Environmental health issues are essentially cross-sectoral, and the conferences bring together different stakeholders to take decisions, working with and across ministries, and involving intergovernmental and international organizations and civil society organizations.

Reduce indoor air pollution

In low- and middle-income countries, preventive measures include improved cooking devices and practices, alternative fuels, placing kitchen separate from the house, avoiding smoke and reducing need for fire, as well as better ventilation of dwellings.

Improved stoves and stove maintenance reduce indoor air pollution and exposure (*399*). In Xuanwei, China, the incidence of COPD decreased markedly after household coal stoves were improved (*400*). Programmes aiming to improve stoves need to obtain wider acceptance and uptake of culturally acceptable and feasible alternatives to the high-exposure cooking stoves currently being used by most people worldwide.

Linkages between household energy technology, indoor air pollution and greenhouse gas emissions have become increasingly important in understanding the local and global environmental and health effects of domestic energy use. Transition from biomass fuels to gas and kerosene would delay several million deaths (*303*). Reducing the use of solid fuels is also economically important and should improve ecosystem stability, since the inefficient use of fuel wood is considered one of the important causes of deforestation (*401*). The social, cultural, economic, technological and environmental implications of each intervention strategy, beyond its impact on exposure reduction, should be monitored (www.who.int/indoorair) and anticipated (*402*). The division of labor, gender relations, and the decision-making process in the household all need to be considered (*401*). Experience gained from projects to introduce improved stoves highlights the importance of involving women in decision making that directly involves their lives (*403*). Home ventilation needs to be improved. In a study in Guatemala, the prevalence of all the symptoms of asthma and severe asthma were higher in children from households that used open fires compared to those using improved stoves with chimneys (*404*).

Strategies to reduce the negative health and environmental effects of solid fuels (www.who.int/heli/risks) include:

- Shifting from solid fuels to cleaner energy technologies, and pricing smokeless fuel competitively to encourage substitution.
- Improving the design of stoves and ventilation systems.
- Raising public awareness of the health risks of indoor air pollution.

In high-income countries, the right to breathe healthy air in dwellings was recognized as a fundamental right by WHO in 2000. The Towards Healthy Air in Dwellings in Europe (THADE) project has been promoted by the European Federation of Asthma and Airways Diseases Patients' Associations (EFA) with the support of the European Commission. The aims of the THADE project are to:

- Produce maps of pollutants in European dwellings.
- Review the data related to exposure to air pollution in dwellings, and to their health effects, particularly as regards allergies, asthma and other chronic respiratory diseases.
- Review cost-effective measures and technology to improve air quality in dwellings.
- Review legislation and guidelines on air pollution and air quality in dwellings.
- Recommend an integrated strategy that defines appropriate indoor air quality policies for implementation in Europe.

The following actions will help to prevent the adverse effects of poor air quality in dwellings:

- Improve ventilation.
- Improve cleaning methods and housing hygiene.
- Avoid wall-to-wall carpeting.
- Control moisture to prevent the accumulation of mould.
- Control the sources of pollution, e.g. tobacco smoke, and emissions from buildings and consumer products.

Avoid allergens

In theory, allergies could possibly be prevented at three levels (*50, 393*). *Primary prevention* takes place before there is any evidence of allergy, in subjects exposed to known risk factors. Because allergy sensitization can occur early in life (*405, 406*), much of the focus of primary prevention will be on perinatal interventions. To date, however, there is no proven effective measure for primary prevention. Research is ongoing, and it is hoped that effective primary prevention strategies will be found. *Secondary prevention* is employed after risk factors have induced an effect, but before there is any clinical evidence of allergy (e.g. primary sensitization to allergens without asthma or rhinitis without asthma). Secondary preventive measures have been tested, but draw doubtful conclusions. *Tertiary prevention* involves the avoidance of risk factors when an allergy is established. Tertiary prevention should be introduced early to prevent long-term consequences of the allergy, which may be intractable even with total avoidance of the risk factor. Although complete avoidance of allergens in high altitude was found to improve allergic asthma, most avoidance measures for mites, animal danders and cockroaches are ineffective (*407*). In inner cities, home-based environmental interventions were found to improve asthma (*408*). More data are needed to establish general strategies for tertiary prevention of allergic asthma.

Prevent occupational chronic respiratory diseases

Occupational chronic respiratory diseases represent, in high–income countries, as well as in low- and middle-income countries, a public health problem with substantial economic implications. Preventing such diseases is therefore extremely important. Given its global mandate, WHO has launched the WHO Global Occupational Health Programme (http://www.who.int/oeh/index.html). Several initiatives have also been launched at governmental level for the prevention of occupational asthma, for example in France (http://www.sante.gouv.fr) on 28 January 2002 and in the United Kingdom (http://www.hse.gov.uk/condocs) on 10 October 2001. Labour unions are deeply involved in the management and prevention of occupational asthma. The three levels of prevention, mentioned before, apply.

Exposure limits are the basis of primary prevention. In the case of occupational asthma, the single most significant determinant is the level of exposure (*340*). For crystalline silica dust, the threshold limit values – time weighted average (TLV-TWA) levels of exposure should not exceed 0.05 to 0.1 mg/m^3 (*409*). A TLV-TWA of 0.5 mg/m^3 has been suggested for flour dust. Maximum exposure to isocyanates should not exceed 5 part per billion at any time.

Exposure to silica dust and agents causing occupational asthma should be reduced by adequate environmental controls and respiratory protection at work. Positive pressure masks have been developed that allow for the complete avoidance of harmful inhalants.

For asbestos exposure, the recommendations are less straightforward. Asbestos has been banned in many countries, principally because of the risk of mesothelioma, a cancer of the pleura. Clearly, spray-on procedures using asbestos fibres and applications of crocidolite asbestos should be banned. A programme should take into account the cost of substitutes to industrializing countries, in particular water-poor countries. For instance, an exception to the ban could be made for certain applications such as the manufacture of water pipes for their burgeoning cities.

If primary prevention is not feasible, then the emphasis has to be on the secondary and tertiary prevention of occupational chronic respiratory diseases. It is of great importance to diagnose the disease early and propose a management plan. Early recognition of occupational chronic respiratory diseases is an essential step in preventing the onset of severe persistent disease which could progress even after the occupational agent has been removed. If exposure continues, symptoms are likely to become increasingly severe (*410, 411*). Once chronic respiratory diseases are established, progression of the disease and asthma exacerbations may be triggered by other agents, such as tobacco smoke, cold air and exercise. If people are removed from exposure to the substance causing chronic respiratory diseases as soon as they start to develop symptoms, they are more likely to make a complete recovery than if the exposure continues. In the case of occupational asthma, early signs are rhinitis and non-specific bronchial hyper-responsiveness. When exposure continues, symptoms of chronic respiratory diseases become increasingly severe and may be permanent.

Comprehensive approach for occupational chronic respiratory diseases prevention

Smoking and tuberculosis are major co-factors in the development and severity of occupational chronic respiratory diseases, necessitating a comprehensive approach to address smoking and tuberculosis in occupational settings (*38, 334, 335*). Individuals with tuberculosis scars in their lungs and smokers who have sub-clinical COPD may be more susceptible than others to developing chronic respiratory diseases when exposed to additional respiratory risk factors.

GARD's efforts will be directed towards facilitating and supporting efforts by countries to draw up and implement an indoors tobacco smoking ban, an action plan to control indoor air pollution, a policy on allergy prevention, and a strategy to prevent occupational chronic respiratory diseases. The success of GARD's efforts will be measured in terms of:

- Increased number of countries with an indoors tobacco smoking ban facilitated by GARD.
- Increased number of countries with an action plan facilitated by GARD to prevent other forms of indoor air pollution.
- Increased number of countries with policies on allergy prevention facilitated by GARD.
- Increased number of countries with an occupational strategy facilitated by GARD.

21. Improve Diagnosis of Chronic Respiratory Diseases and Respiratory Allergies

KEY MESSAGES

- **In all countries, chronic respiratory diseases are underdiagnosed.**
- **There is a need for early diagnosis of chronic respiratory diseases in order to reduce the severity of disease and disability.**
- **Ideally, low-cost and effective spirometry should be accessible to all. However, at present, the use of spirometry for all patients at risk cannot be recommended as it would require resources that are not readily available in many low-income countries.**

To improve the diagnosis of chronic respiratory diseases and respiratory allergies, it is necessary to consider:

- Target population (whole population, groups at risk, individuals).
- Stages of disease (early disease, established disease, disability).
- Importance of risk factors inducing the disease (low risk or high risk).
- Level of affluence of the country.

This chapter focuses primarily on asthma and chronic obstructive pulmonary disease. GARD suggests the use of a symptom-driven approach to initially develop a "syndromic" definition of chronic respiratory disease.

Chronic respiratory diseases are under-diagnosed in all countries, but particularly in low- and middle-income countries. Many patients are not diagnosed until chronic respiratory diseases are severe enough to prevent normal daily activities, including attendance at school or work. Wheezing is often considered to be the expression of an acute infection. The diagnosis of chronic respiratory diseases is delayed, being made only after several exacerbations. There are a limited number of diagnostic tests for the early screening of predisposition to COPD, asthma or allergy. These tests are generally not used correctly to establish preventive measures in groups at risk. Training on the indications for diagnostic testing, and on the use and interpretation of diagnostic tests, is insufficient. Furthermore, in low- and middle-income countries, much medical equipment is not in use because of a lack of maintenance or spare parts, because it is too sophisticated, or simply because the health personnel do not know how to use it.

GARD will develop recommendations to countries on how to:

- Provide simple, available and affordable diagnostic tools for chronic respiratory diseases and respiratory allergies, using a stepwise approach adapted to different health needs, services and resources.
- Provide evidence-based training for health-care professionals on diagnosis of these conditions.

Box 7 Diagnosis: potential synergies

Diagnostic algorithms developed as part of the Practical Approach to Lung health (PAL).

Occupational health policies for diagnosis.

Strategy to assist national health authorities in the selection, procurement, use and disposal of high-quality medical devices that meet their particular needs (www.who.int/medical_devices/en/) as part of public health policy. A chronic respiratory diseases module will be developed by GARD.

Global Alliance on Healthcare Technology: an initiative of WHO and the World Bank to propose practical solutions to the major problems facing low- and middle-income countries regarding health technology.

Other recommendations for diagnosis:

American Academy of Allergy, Asthma and Immunology (AAAAI) and American College of Allergy, Asthma and Immunology (ACAAI): practice parameters on asthma and rhinitis (*412*).

Allergic Rhinitis and its Impact on Asthma (ARIA): diagnosis of allergy and rhinitis (*51*).

American Thoracic Society/European Respiratory Society (ATS/ERS): standards for the diagnosis and treatment of COPD (*106*). Recently a landmark for the implementation of pulmonary function tests has been achieved through the ATS/ERS standards, published as a series of articles in 2005 (*416–421*), setting a benchmark that will facilitate the manufacturing and use of homogeneous instruments, thereby reducing technical variability and promoting the widespread use of functional evaluations.

European Academy of Allergology and Clinical Immunology (EAACI): position paper on skin tests (*422*).

Global Initiative for Asthma (GINA): diagnosis of asthma (*50*).

Global Initiative for Chronic Obstructive Pulmonary Disease (GOLD): diagnosis of COPD (*107*).

International Primary Care Airways Group (IPAG): guidelines for the diagnosis of chronic respiratory diseases (www.theipcrg.org/guidelines/ipag_backgrounder.php).

International Primary Care Respiratory Group (IPCRG): guidelines for the diagnosis of chronic respiratory diseases (*423, 424*).

What will GARD do to improve the diagnosis of chronic respiratory diseases?

The aims of GARD's activities are to:

- Reduce the under-diagnosis of chronic respiratory diseases.
- Advocate for early diagnosis of chronic respiratory diseases.
- Ensure that all patients with chronic respiratory diseases have access to affordable diagnostic tests.
- Develop training programmes for health-care workers on diagnostic testing, covering indications for carrying out diagnostic tests, and the use and interpretation of results.

The diagnosis of chronic respiratory diseases is based on a stepwise investigation (Figure 23).

- The first diagnostic step is a simple questionnaire to assess clinical presentation. A questionnaire and an **examination of the patient** are, however, incomplete predictors of airflow limitation.

- The second diagnostic step is a **simple lung-function measurement** using spirometry. This will improve the sensitivity of the diagnosis evaluation and the assessment of severity of the disease. Accurate diagnosis is important because treatment for asthma and COPD differ. Additionally, recording a correct diagnosis will improve the validity of epidemiological studies (*425*).

- The third diagnostic step consists of other tests, including **full pulmonary function tests, oxymetry and allergy tests** (*426*). Such tests will be performed, when needed, to improve the diagnosis further, refine the assessment of severity, follow up patients, and give an insight into risk factors.

Figure 23 Diagnosis of chronic respiratory diseases based on a stepwise investigation

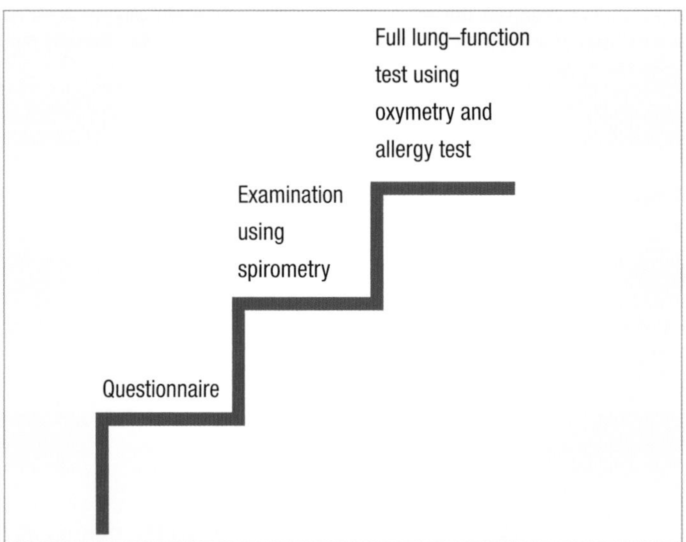

One of the major goals of GARD is to ensure that pulmonary function testing, under the second diagnostic step, is available and accessible to all patients. At present, however, the use of spirometry for all patients at risk cannot be recommended, as it would require the testing of a large number of individuals and would involve tremendous costs and taking up too much of health-workers' time.

Moreover, low-cost, efficient spirometers still need to be selected. The training of health-care workers also represents a large task. A working group of the Forum of International Respiratory Societies (FIRS) is currently investigating this problem, and GARD will use its recommendations.

It is unclear whether lung-function testing would induce behavioral changes, including smoking cessation (*427*).

Ensuring the availability and accessibility of simple allergy tests is another of GARD's goals for the second diagnostic step. The use of a validated and standard tool for diagnosis of atopy will make comparisons between populations more reliable. This is crucial for identification of risk factors and to test interventions.

GARD will produce the following deliverables:

- Manual on the diagnosis of chronic respiratory diseases, including a questionnaire and guidance on simple lung-function measurement.
- Manual on allergy diagnosis in low- and middle-income countries.

What will GARD do to improve the diagnosis of asthma and COPD at country level?

Asthma

- The Global Initiative for Asthma (GINA) (*50*) and the United States National Asthma Education and Prevention Programme (NAEPP) guidelines (*428*) advocate the measurement of symptoms and lung function to diagnose asthma, and medication requirements to assess severity. Although this approach is feasible and very accurate (*429*), it is, however, underused (*430, 431*). Furthermore, as it is only feasible in patients over 5 years old, the diagnosis of asthma in infants and young children is still a problem (*432*).
- Simple questionnaires can differentiate between asthma and COPD (*433–435*).
- When asthma is diagnosed and the treatment established, it is essential to monitor follow-up. A shift in the paradigm of follow-up has occurred within the past 5 years. Many guidelines now recommend assessing the control of asthma, and basing management on current therapies and quality of control (*436*). Control can be assessed by asking patients a few simple questions about night-time symptoms, daytime symptoms, activities of daily life, needs for rescue medication, and frequency of unscheduled visits to a doctor or hospital for an asthma exacerbation (*437*). Various instruments have been proposed and some have been validated, including the Royal College of Physicians' Asthma Control Test (*438*) or Asthma Control Questionnaire (*439*).
- Additionally, measures of lung function may be used to follow up patients (*440*). Monitoring peak expiratory flow (PEF) is an important and affordable clinical tool in the emergency department and hospital, and for a few patients is useful in the home (*441*).

At national level, GARD will promote the implementation of action plans that:

- Provide simple questionnaires for asthma screening.

- Educate health-care providers in the use of the questionnaires.
- Increase the availability and accessibility of pulmonary function tests for all patients.
- Improve the follow-up of patients, by means of control assessment.
- Develop simple and affordable allergy tests.
- Assure the availability and accessibility of inhaled corticosteroids and bronchodilators.

Chronic obstructive pulmonary disease

The classification of disease severity into four stages for the management of COPD is largely symptom-driven (106). This staging, as laid out by WHO (http://www.who.int/respiratory/en/), "is a pragmatic approach aimed at practical implementation and should only be regarded as an educational tool, and a very general indication of the approach to management". It implies that the leading principle for diagnosis is clinical presentation, rather than the presence of risk factors such as cigarette smoke and exposure to particles. Admittedly, the relationship between degree of airflow limitation and the presence of symptoms is imperfect.

The use of simple questionnaires has been advocated for use at primary care (*434, 442–445*) or referral level (*446*).

The GOLD guidelines (*107*) base the diagnosis of COPD on a history of exposure to risk factors and the "presence of airflow limitation that is not fully reversible, with or without the presence of symptoms". Lung-function tests should be performed for airflow limitation, even in the absence of dyspnea. COPD can be diagnosed on the basis of case history, and physical, and laboratory data, even if spirometry is not available *(107*).

Spirometry is the gold standard for the diagnosis and assessment of COPD, as it is the most reproducible, standardized and objective way of measuring airflow limitation. Clearly, spirometry could be used in primary care, provided that adequate resources, training and quality control were available (*447*). However, in most primary health care centres in the world, spirometry is not available. The threshold $FEV_1/FVC < 70\%$ has been proposed to confirm the presence of an airflow limitation that is not fully reversible. It is questionable, however, whether this measurement should be advocated, since chronic severe asthma might present with an irreversible component, and the intensive use of combined bronchodilator drugs might induce reversibility in COPD patients.

The measurement of lung function should therefore be advocated for the diagnosis of COPD in symptomatic patients, complementing clinical information and identifying those with severe disease. There is insufficient evidence to recommend lung-function screening for populations at risk, and there is insufficient evidence to determine whether the early detection of COPD by lung function measurement alone would improve the prognosis.

22. Control Chronic Respiratory Diseases and Allergies by Increasing Drug Accessibility

KEY MESSAGES

- **An integrated approach to the prevention, diagnosis and management of chronic respiratory diseases, as proposed in the WHO Practical Approach to Lung Health (PAL) and the WHO Practical Approach to Lung Health in South Africa (PALSA Plus) is recommended by GARD as suitable for primary care in low- and middle-income countries.**
- **In high-income countries, disease-specific approaches may be more appropriate.**
- **Chronic respiratory diseases in childhood and adolescence need a specific attention.**
- **In all countries, the control of occupational chronic respiratory diseases is a priority.**
- **Access to and affordability of diagnostics and drugs are essential.**
- **GARD action plans should be tailored to each country's needs, priorities, health services and resources.**

In all countries:

- Chronic respiratory diseases are unrecognized and under-treated.
- Education of health-care providers needs to be improved.
- Integration of care for chronic respiratory diseases between primary and referral levels is essential for optimal management of these chronic diseases.

In low- and middle-income countries:

- Most patients with asthma or COPD receive treatment only during exacerbations, rather than benefiting from continuous care.
- Drugs are often unavailable or not affordable.
- In low-resource settings, putting evidence into practice requires context-specific and user-friendly formats, such as algorithms (*21*).

What will GARD do?

GARD will work to improve the control of chronic respiratory diseases and related allergies through:

- The development, validation and implementation of simple and affordable approaches.
- The training of health professionals appropriate for each country's needs, priorities, health-care systems and resources.

Action plans need to be tailored to low-, middle- and high-income countries or regions within countries (Figure 24). In areas with a high burden of communicable diseases and functioning primary health-care centres, approaches such as the WHO Practical Approach to Lung Health (PAL) model will be promoted. In areas with a high prevalence of HIV infection, approaches such as PAL in South Africa (PALSA Plus) will be promoted.

Models of prevention and care for chronic respiratory diseases in middle- and high-income countries will be different. They will target asthma, rhinitis, COPD, occupational lung diseases and pulmonary hypertension. Approaches will be developed from available management plans and international guidelines, according to specific country needs.

Key aspects of GARD action plans will be:

- To ensure the availability and accessibility of drugs for patients with chronic respiratory diseases in each treatment setting.
- To assist in knowledge translation strategies for the training of health-care workers in the management of chronic respiratory diseases, particularly the control of occupational chronic respiratory diseases and pulmonary hypertension.

Figure 24 Goals of chronic respiratory disease control, according to the income–level of the country

In high–income countries

- patients can receive adequate diagnosis and treatment
- but they are insufficiently diagnosed and treated
- a disease–specific approach is needed
- the goals of GARD are to better diagnose, treat and educate patients.

In upper–middle–income countries

- few patients can receive adequate diagnosis and treatment
- the first goal of GARD is to reduce under–diagnosis
- the second goal of GARD is to provide accessible and affordable treatment for all patients
- a syndromic approach (PAL) is needed in many places.

In lower–middle and low–income countries

- very few patients can receive adequate diagnosis and treatment
- the first goal of GARD is to reduce under–diagnosis
- the second goal of GARD is to provide accessible and affordable treatment for all patients
- a syndromic approach (PAL) is needed in most places.

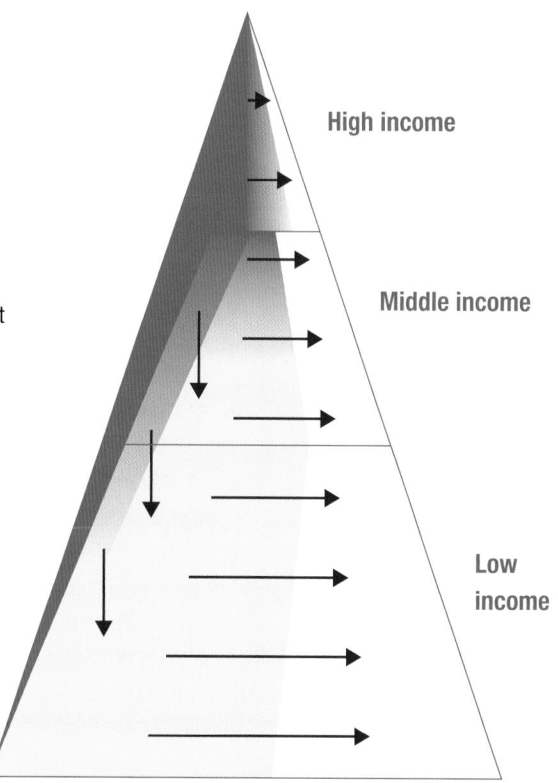

The arrows indicate the goals of GARD

■ Control by disease-specific approach
Control by syndromic approach
□ No control

Box 8 Control of chronic respiratory diseases: potential synergies

To promote synergy among existing WHO and non-WHO activities, avoid duplication and overlap, and improve coordination in implementing GARD Country activities, GARD Basket will be developed, where existing WHO and non-WHO programmes will be offered to every country interested in a CD-Rom.

WHO activities

ILO/WHO Global Campaign for the Elimination of Silicosis

WHO occupational health (www.who.int/occupational_health/en/)

WHO Practical Approach to Lung Health (PAL) and the WHO Practical Approach to Lung Health in South Africa (PALSAPlus) (*448, 449*).

Other activities

National programmes for asthma and COPD (see Table 19).

Box 9 The WHO Practical Approach to Lung Health (PAL) and the WHO Practical Approach to Lung Health in South Africa (PALSA) Plus

The Practical Approach to Lung Health (PAL) strategy has been developed by WHO to improve the quality of tuberculosis (TB) diagnosis, increase TB case detection among respiratory patients, and improve the diagnosis and care of patients with common respiratory diseases (*448, 449*). Thus, PAL forms part of both the Stop TB (*376*) and the GARD strategies. In settings where the prevalence of HIV is high, PAL may be adapted to assist clinicians in the primary care management of patients with HIV/AIDS.

Rationale for the development of the Practical Approach to Lung Health

Globally, respiratory conditions rank first or second among reasons for patients' seeking care at primary health-care facilities and account for up to one third of patients seen at these facilities. Tuberculosis is diagnosed in only a small proportion (≤ 2%) of these patients, and for other common respiratory diseases, facilities and guidelines for the correct diagnosis and management are often non-standardized, empirical and inadequate, resulting in under-recognition of certain diseases (such as asthma and COPD) or inappropriate treatment (for example, over-use of antibiotics). Since symptoms of cough and breathlessness are common to most major respiratory diseases, the PAL approach is to use these symptoms to recognize potential respiratory disease (including tuberculosis), and to guide correct diagnosis and management through use of an integrated standardized evidence-based guideline tailored to the needs of front-line clinicians in each region or country setting.

Features of the Practical Approach to Lung Health strategy

The PAL strategy is the syndromic diagnosis and integrated management of patients with respiratory symptoms. It focuses on patients aged 5 years and over in the primary health care setting. Respiratory diseases to which the strategy accords priority include :

- Tuberculosis.
- Acute respiratory infections, particularly pneumonia.
- Chronic respiratory diseases, mainly asthma and COPD.

The PAL strategy aims to improve the quality of care of every patient, seeking care for respiratory symptoms and improving the efficiency of the health services caring for such patients. The PAL approach needs to be

CONTINUED ON NEXT PAGE

BOX 9 (CONTINUED)

adapted in each country to accommodate and conform to national health policies and health priorities, and to be based on epidemiological realities and specificities, as well as on the health resources available within each country.

Components of the Practical Approach to Lung Health strategy

Key components of the PAL strategy are standardization of diagnosis, management and follow-up of respiratory patients through the adaptation and development of integrated clinical practice guidelines, and coordination between the primary care (first level) health facilities and referral levels within the district health system. In each country, the latter requires the coordinated involvement of many elements within health care services, particularly those responsible for primary health care, the essential drugs programme, the national tuberculosis programme, the HIV/AIDS programme and health management information systems.

Implementing the Practical Approach to Lung Health strategy at country level

The development of the PAL strategy involves the following steps:

- Political commitment from national health authorities to adapt, develop and implement PAL.
- Formation of a national working group, comprising all key stakeholders in health care, to adapt, develop, plan, implement and fund the PAL strategy.
- Assessment of the health care environment, including national health priorities, health infrastructure and resources, funding procedures and institutional mechanisms that might facilitate the development and implementation of PAL, and potential barriers to the development and implementation of PAL at each level of the health-care chain.
- Adaptation of the PAL clinical practice guidelines and training material.
- Identification of pilot sites that can be used to audit the impact of the PAL intervention, bearing in mind that the audit should cover improvements in quality of care and health outcomes, as well as improvements in disease management and their outcomes.
- Development, with the relevant health authority, of a multi-year and stepwise plan (including costs) for wider implementation of PAL.
- Exploration, with national health authorities, of potential sources of funding for rolling out PAL (possible sources include government, regional administration, health sector reform funds, donors, or bilateral or multilateral cooperative agreements).
- Implementation of PAL should preferably be led by a clearly identified unit under the leadership of a ministerial entity such as the national tuberculosis programme or primary health care department.
- Establishing a monitoring and evaluation system to assess the quality and performance of PAL activities.

Potential impact of the Practical Approach to Lung Health strategy at the country level

The development and implementation of PAL is under way in approximately 30 countries and some results are already available (*22, 375*). Experience to date suggests that PAL is likely to:

- Improve tuberculosis detection and the quality of tuberculosis diagnosis (*22*).
- Strengthen the integration of tuberculosis control services within primary health care.
- Improve the diagnosis and care of patients with other priority respiratory diseases through the provision of an integrated health-care package (*22*).

CONTINUED ON NEXT PAGE

BOX 9 (CONTINUED)

- **Improve the referral system for patients with respiratory conditions requiring higher levels of care.**
- **Increase primary health care attendance for respiratory conditions.**
- **Help national health authorities cope with the health sector reform through standardization of respiratory care and identification of the required health resources.**
- **Improve planning and health resource management.**
- **Reduce drug prescription, particularly antibiotics and adjuvant drugs.**
- **Improve the quality of drug prescription for chronic respiratory disease patients.**
- **Reduce the average cost of drug prescription per respiratory patient in some settings.**

The Practical Approach to Lung Health in high-HIV prevalence countries (PALSA Plus)

In countries with a high burden of HIV, the PAL strategy may be adapted further to include the diagnosis and care of patients with HIV-related diseases and infections, even at the primary care level (*22*). Whereas in most countries, HIV treatment, especially the administration of antiretroviral drugs, is viewed as a specialized service, in the worst affected countries, the majority of care is provided at primary care level, in particular for respiratory infections or complications (upper and lower respiratory tract infections, *Pneumocystis* pneumonia, tuberculosis). One such adaptation, PALSA Plus, has been piloted and introduced in some regions of South Africa (*22*).

HIV-care offered (or potentially offered) by PALSA Plus includes:

- **Syndromic diagnosis of common and opportunistic infections, with where necessary the early introduction of antibiotics and referral to the next level of care.**
- **Voluntary confidential counselling and testing for HIV infection.**
- **Post-exposure prophylaxis with antiretroviral treatment.**
- **Monitoring of drug adherence for tuberculosis, isoniazid, prophylaxis, co-trimoxazole prophylaxis, and antiretroviral treatment drugs.**
- **Collection of routine monitoring specimens (CD4 counts, lactic acid levels and other safety investigations, as well as sputum examination for the success of tuberculosis treatment).**

GARD will produce the following deliverables:

Asthma

An asthma action plan has already been proposed by the ministry of health in countries such as Brazil, Finland (*450*), France (*451*), Portugal, and the United States (www.nhlbi.nih.gov/guidelines/asthma). The results of the action plans are generally impressive. They have reduced morbidity and mortality attributable to asthma in high-income (*58*) and low- and middle-income countries as well as in deprived areas (*60, 75, 76*). In Finland, however, the plan had no effect on the prevalence of the disease, which is still increasing.

GARD's activities are based on available guidelines, updated with the latest knowledge on asthma. In particular, treatment should no longer be based only on severity (*50, 452*), but also on control (*436*) and treatment needs (*453*).

Many guidelines are available for the management of asthma. These include GINA (*50*), NAEPP (*454, 455*), ARIA (*51, 456*), IPAG (www.theipcrg.org/guidelines/ipag_backgrounder.php), IPCRG (*457–461*), BTS (*462*) and other national guidelines (*436*). For low- and middle-income countries, the International Union against Tuberculosis and Lung Diseases has developed a guide for asthma management focusing on the WHO list of essential drugs (*23*).

Occupational asthma is discussed on page 51.

GARD expects that its efforts will produce the following results:

- Maintenance of capacity for school and work, and functional capacity of people with asthma.
- Improvement of health status.
- Reduction in hospitalizations and stays in an intensive care unit – these results cannot be demonstrated in many low- and middle-income countries where patients are not hospitalized for asthma or where hospitalizations or visits to emergency departments are not recorded (*13, 59*).
- Reduction in asthma deaths – this result cannot be demonstrated in many low- and middle-income countries where mortality rates are not recorded (*13, 59*).
- Optimization of management effectiveness.

GARD will promote national action plans that follow the guidance below.

Improve surveillance and awareness of asthma and its risk factors. Patient education programmes should increase awareness, and eliminate social stigma and misconception in the community regarding asthma. Knowledge about the prevailing perception in the community would be the first step in achieving this (*463*). A particular effort is needed in schools, where nurses should be able to recognize undiagnosed asthma and improve the implementation of asthma management plans (*464–466*).

Start early effective treatment according to the patient's control of asthma and current medications, win the patient's confidence and follow up the efficacy of the treatment. The goal is asthma control (*436, 462, 467–470*). Achieving asthma control reduces exacerbations (*471, 472*). Early controller therapy may be important for the optimal management of asthma (*473*). Guidelines for the treatment of asthma should be tailored to the country's needs, health system, and drug availability and accessibility. It has been found, in practice, that guidelines for asthma are not well implemented, partly because they are complex and, possibly, because treatment based on severity may not meet the patient's needs. Asthma care in general practice should be promoted to reduce barriers (*474, 475*). At follow-up, if the patient is not controlled, it is important to check compliance and inhalation technique.

Recognize and treat acute exacerbations early. Asthma mortality continues to be a serious global problem in many parts of the world, and several risk factors have been identified for fatal or near-fatal exacerbations (*476*). Early identification and treatment of an acute exacerbation is effective and may prevent death.

Consider asthma and rhinitis in the same patient. Most patients with asthma have rhinitis, and many patients with rhinitis have asthma. Patients with persistent allergic rhinitis should be evaluated for asthma by taking a history of symptoms, chest examination and, where necessary, the assessment of airflow obstruction before and after bronchodilator. Patients with asthma should be appropriately evaluated (taking a history and doing a physical examination) for rhinitis. In terms of efficacy and safety, a combined strategy should ideally be used to treat the upper and lower airway diseases (*51*).

Educate the patient, preferably providing a written management plan. Non-adherence to treatment advice is common in asthma and accounts for a significant proportion of morbidity. Asthma education and self-management are recommended. Educational programmes that offer information about asthma but not self-management skills are not very effective (*477, 478*). Training programmes that enable people to adjust their medication using a written plan appear to be more effective (*479*); but further results are needed to fully assess the value of such plans (*480*).

Educate health-care professionals. This is an essential step, since the use of appropriate methods depends on appropriate training (481). Educational programmes should be targeted to the needs of the country or region concerned, and should be assessed.

Chronic obstructive pulmonary disease

A COPD action plan has already been proposed by the ministry of health in countries such as Finland (*482*), France (*483*) and Portugal.

GARD supports action plans updated with the latest knowledge on COPD, such as the ATS/ERS (*106*), GOLD (*107, 484*), NICE (*485, 486*), IPAG (www.theipcrg.org/guidelines/ipag_backgrounder.php), IPCRG (*432, 461, 462*) or other national guidelines (*482, 487–492*). Guidelines should be locally adapted by a working group of health professionals, and should be agreed between the ministry of health, WHO and the GARD Country Coordinator.

GARD expects that its activities will produce the following tangible results in terms of the prevention and control of COPD:

- Decrease in the occurrence of COPD in the general population, in particular by reducing risk factors and by improving home, work and school environment.
- Diagnosis of patients in early stages of COPD.
- Maintenance of capacity for work and functional capacity of patients with COPD.
- Improvement of the health status of patients with COPD.

- Reduction in the percentage of patients with moderate to severe COPD.

- Cessation of deterioration – or decline in the rate of deterioration – of pulmonary function.

- Reduction in complications of the disease and deaths.

- Optimization of management effectiveness.

GARD will support national action plans that follow the approach below.

Improve the surveillance and awareness of COPD and its risk factors, in the general population and in key groups. COPD, even more than asthma, is under-diagnosed and under-recognized (*494, 495*), in particular in low- and middle-income countries. General awareness of COPD in the community is extremely poor. A particular effort is needed in key groups (smokers, occupational settings), where health-care workers should be able to recognize undiagnosed COPD. National campaigns are needed to promote the awareness of COPD and its risk factors.

Promote preventive measures. The primary prevention of COPD in the general population, and the secondary and tertiary prevention of COPD in key groups, are important worldwide, particularly in low- and middle-income countries. Preventive measures include:

- Prevention and cessation of smoking – morbidity (*496*), mortality (*497*) and decline in lung function are reduced in patients with early COPD who stop smoking (*498, 499*).

- Reduction in indoor air pollution.

- Reduction in work-related pollutants.

- Reduction of outdoor air pollutants.

- Prevention of recurrent respiratory infections in children.

Promote early diagnosis and active treatment, in particular among smokers and people who are exposed to risk factors. COPD is usually asymptomatic or presents few symptoms for many years before it is diagnosed. Pharmacological treatment should follow established guidelines (*106, 107, 500, 501*).

Recognize and treat exacerbations early. COPD is often associated with exacerbations of symptoms which may be life-threatening (*117, 502, 503*). COPD is often undiagnosed and may be revealed during an exacerbation, which may be severe. Early diagnosis and management of exacerbations can reduce hospitalizations and may also improve the natural course of COPD (*504*). Influenza vaccination can prevent the occurrence of exacerbations (*505*).

Start physical exercise and rehabilitation early; this should be planned individually and implemented as part of the treatment. The principal goal of rehabilitation is to reduce symptoms, so as to improve quality of life and increase physical and emotional participation in everyday activities (*506–510*). Rehabilitation may only be cost-effective in patients with severe COPD (*511*).

Initiate oxygen therapy in patients with chronic respiratory failure. Oxygen therapy has been shown to increase survival among patients with chronic respiratory failure. Treatment should be in line with published recommendations (*106, 107, 512, 513*).

Monitor follow-up and considerer co-morbidities. There should be regular follow-up visits, and therapy should be adjusted appropriately as the disease progresses. It is important to consider concomitant conditions, such as bronchial carcinoma (*221, 514*), tuberculosis, sleep apnea syndrome (*515*), left-heart failure (*214*) and loss of bone density (*106, 107, 516*).

Educate the patient and improve guided self-care. Although patient education does not improve exercise performance or lung function, it may play a role in improving skills, ability to cope with illness, and health status (*106, 107, 517*).

Educate health care professionals.

Advocate for more scientific research.

Occupational lung diseases

About 45% of the world's population and 58% of the population over 10 years of age belong to the global workforce. Their work sustains the economic and material basis of society, which is critically dependent on their working capacity. Thus occupational health and the well-being of working people are crucial prerequisites for productivity and are of the utmost importance for overall socioeconomic and sustainable development (*518*).

GARD expects that its efforts will produce the following results:

- Reduction of risk factors at a level which they will not cause chronic respiratory diseases (or sensitization).
- Maintenance of capacity for work.
- Reduction in severe occupational chronic respiratory diseases.
- Reduction in deaths attributable to occupational chronic respiratory diseases.
- Optimization of management effectiveness.

GARD will support national action plans that follow the approach outlined below.

Improve the surveillance and awareness of occupational lung diseases. Within occupational settings, it is important to investigate the information provided by health-care workers and employees in order to improve the detection of early onset of occupational lung disease. There is a great need to develop intervention strategies through adequate surveillance programmes in high-risk workplaces (*519*). In South Africa, the Surveillance of Work-related and Occupational Respiratory Diseases in South Africa (SORDSA) registry was established in 1996 to provide systematic information on occupational respiratory diseases (*520, 521*). This registry can be used as a model for other low- and middle-income countries.

Prevent exposure.

- Action should be taken by all employers and employees before exposure occurs, according to available recommendations.
- Exposure to asbestos dust should be avoided through substitution by alternative products. Exceptions (for example, pipes to ensure safe water and sanitation) should be considered for low-income countries with poor water supplies. .
- Exposure to silica dust should be reduced to comply with international standards, such as the International Labour Organization/WHO Global Campaign for the Elimination of Silicosis (*522*).
- Exposure to agents that may cause occupational asthma or COPD should be reduced.
- Use of positive pressure masks should be promoted for workers exposed to silica dust and other airborne particles.

Promote early diagnosis and active treatment. Occupational lung diseases should be confirmed by objective evidence. Chest radiographs are essential to confirm diseases caused by inorganic dust. International standards for interpreting chest radiographs should be adhered to. The diagnosis of occupational asthma is too often based only on a history of work-related symptoms and not sufficiently on objective evidence (*523*). Also, the diagnosis is generally made too late, resulting in the perpetuation of asthma despite termination of exposure. The long-term sequelae of occupational asthma can be avoided if the affected workers are removed early from exposure.

- Even though their specificity is low, chest radiographs should be carried out routinely and periodically in workers exposed to asbestos and silica dust, in order to detect lung fibrosis (*524*).
- In settings where workers are exposed to risk factors, they should be screened for early signs of sensitization, such as rhinitis (*519*), cough and asthma.
- If suspected, occupational asthma should be confirmed by objective testing (*523, 525*).
- In workplaces that may contribute to the onset of COPD, workers should be monitored at regular intervals, using spirometry.

- Once the diagnosis is confirmed, affected workers should be removed completely from exposure to risk factors, and adequate social rehabilitation programmes should be offered. A delay in ending exposure to risk may result in severe intractable chronic respiratory disease. Appropriate treatment of chronic respiratory disease should be initiated early.

Monitor the long-term follow-up, even in patients who are completely removed from risk factors. Unfortunately, many patients with occupational chronic respiratory diseases are diagnosed at a late stage. Their symptoms may not decrease; they may even worsen. In some cases, such as in patients with silicosis and asbestosis, chronic respiratory disease may occur several years after exposure to risk factors has ended. It is therefore important to follow up the patients regularly for several years after the diagnosis of chronic respiratory diseases even after exposure cessation.

Educate the patient and improve guided self-care.

Educate health-care professionals, in particular those working in the occupational setting. Health workers need to ask pertinent work-related questions to workers exposed to risk factors, in order to initiate timely investigations and referral (*526*).

Provide compensation for work loss. Occupational chronic respiratory diseases are often not adequately recognized as a problem in low- and middle-income countries, although their economic consequences are of major importance. In many low- and middle-income countries, occupational diseases are not compensated, and patients continue to work despite suffering from lung diseases of increasing severity.

Pulmonary hypertension

Idiopathic pulmonary arterial hypertension, also known as primary pulmonary hypertension, is very rare. Pulmonary arterial hypertension associated with other conditions, such as COPD, systemic sclerosis, congenital heart diseases, portal hypertension and HIV infection, affects millions of patients around the world. There are wide regional differences in pulmonary hypertension, depending on the cause.

GARD expects that its efforts will produce the following results:

- Increased number of management plans on pulmonary hypertension in high-prevalence areas.
- Maintenance of capacity for work in patients with pulmonary hypertension.
- Reduction in prevalence of intractable pulmonary hypertension and number of associated deaths.

GARD will support national action plans that follow the approach outlined below.

Increase knowledge about the risks for pulmonary hypertension and improve surveillance in high-prevalence areas and among people at risk. Awareness and surveillance of pulmonary hypertension are relevant in areas or populations where there is a high prevalence of schistosomiasis (Brazil, Egypt, South-East Asia, etc.), sickle cell disease or thalassaemia (Africa and in people of African origin worldwide, as well as in people from Mediterranean countries), among people living at high altitudes, and among people suffering from systemic sclerosis, congenital heart diseases, COPD or liver disease.

Promote early diagnosis and active treatment in high-prevalence areas and among people at risk.

- There are no early symptoms of pulmonary hypertension, but the diagnosis should be suspected in patients with increasing dyspnoea on exertion and a known cause of pulmonary hypertension, although lung-function tests may be normal.
- Simple tools help in screening populations at risk (electrocardiogram and chest X-ray).
- Echocardiography-doppler is a more accurate method of screening, allowing a non-invasive measurement of systolic pulmonary arterial pressure. Echocardiography could be performed in regional referral centres.
- A definite diagnosis of pulmonary hypertension requires invasive measurements (right-heart catheterization) in a tertiary referral centres (*263*).
- Much has been learned about pathophysiology, leading to the development of new medications, many of which are quite expensive but improve survival rates (*527*). Low-cost conventional therapy is of interest and includes anticoagulants (warfarin, heparin), calcium antagonists in a minority of patients who respond acutely to a vasodilator challenge (e.g. nifedipine, diltiazem), diuretics, and oxygen therapy (*528*). These low-cost treatments should be available for all patients with pulmonary hypertension.

Give priority to early diagnosis and treatment of all forms of infection in schistosomiasis. This will reduce the risk of pulmonary hypertension.

Box 10 The asthma drug facility initiative: controlling asthma by increasing drug accessibility

To increase the affordability of treatment, the International Union Against Tuberculosis and Lung Disease (the Union) launched a global asthma drug facility initiative to ensure essential good quality drugs for asthma treatment worldwide. This initiative could contribute largely to setting up adequate management of asthma patients in low- and middle-income countries.

Most people with asthma live in low- and middle-income countries and deprived areas. However, access to essential drugs is limited in these regions, often because of prohibitively high prices. Although the disease is common, many patients do not receive an adequate diagnosis and treatment, which exacerbates the condition and leads to additional costs with health resources utilization. A 1998 study found that inhaled beclomethasone was consistently available in only four out of eight countries surveyed (*17*). The cost of inhaled beclomethasone varied more than fivefold, and that of inhaled salbutamol more than threefold. In general, the highest prices were observed in the poorest countries. In all but two countries, the cost of one year of treatment for a case of moderate persistent asthma exceeded the monthly salary of a nurse. In addition, patients did not have any health insurance in six of the countries surveyed. These patients could not be treated with inhaled steroids (*17*).

One of the most important messages of the first World Asthma Meeting, held in 1999, was: “There is a huge need for an international action for making effective asthma therapy available in all countries all over the world” (*529*).

In 2002, another study demonstrated the high cost of inhaled beclomethasone in several countries and the possibility of dramatically decreasing this cost by pooling the purchase of a good quality generic medication (*530*).

In 2003, affordable essential asthma drugs were not reaching patients in low- and middle-income countries. The low affordability of essential asthma drugs remains the main barrier to adequate management of asthma. This has been confirmed by the preliminary results of the Global Asthma Survey on Practice: a study conducted in several countries as an audit in emergency rooms showed that the major factor associated with emergency visits is the low affordability for patients of the drugs used for the long-term treatment of asthma (P Burney, personal communication).

The Global Drug Facility for tuberculosis drugs in 2001 used pooled procurement from pre-qualified producers of anti-tuberculosis drugs, along with other purchasing and supply strategies (*531*). The cost of tuberculosis drugs continues to decrease with the creation of the Global Drug Facility, and an independent evaluation concluded that the Global Drug Facility had been vital for the successful expansion of the DOTS strategy in high-burden countries. Initially, countries received drugs as a grant from the Global Drug Facility, but now direct procurement by countries is becoming more common.

Based on this experience, a similar model has been introduced for the procurement of asthma drugs. The Union’s standardized approach for the management of asthma, which uses only two inhaled medications – steroids and short-acting ß-agonists (*23*) – can be implemented in most low- and middle-income countries if affordable drugs are made available to all patients. The concept of an Asthma Drug Facility, recently proposed by the Union (*532*), could be introduced if the pharmaceutical companies that produce essential asthma drugs could provide these drugs at affordable prices for patients in low- and middle-income countries.

It has been proposed that the Asthma Drug Facility should be organized along the same lines as the Global Drug Facility, which pre-qualifies producers of essential asthma drugs to guarantee quality and obtain the lowest prices. The Asthma Drug Facility would pool procurement for low- and middle-income countries interested in direct procurement. The increased affordability of drugs for patients would rapidly lead to immense health benefits and huge improvements in asthma management in those countries. It would be critical, of course, to also provide technical assistance to these countries regarding asthma management, storage and the distribution of essential asthma drugs of proven good quality.

The rationale and description of the Asthma Drug Facility concept was published in an editorial in 2004 (*532*). The concept was presented at the Union’s Africa Region Conference in February 2004 and prompted positive feedback from colleagues in low- and middle-income countries. The concept was presented at the Union World Conference in November 2004 and 2005 and was supported by several partners including WHO.

23. Paediatric Chronic Respiratory Diseases and Respiratory Allergies

KEY MESSAGES

- **Asthma and rhinitis are the most frequent chronic diseases in children.**
- **Asthma is underdiagnosed and undertreated in children worldwide. A previous specific WHO initiative in the field was not existing.**
- **In many low- and middle-income countries asthma exacerbations in children is a leading cause of admissions and emergency visits.**

Chronic respiratory diseases in children should be considered in the context of low-, middle- and high-income settings (Box 10), and GARD should set short-, medium- and long-term goals.

The most common respiratory problem in children under 14 years of age is acute respiratory distress, usually considered to be of infectious etiology. Respiratory infections differ widely between high-income countries where they are usually mild (*533*), and low- and middle-income countries where they cause an enormous burden and high death rate (*534, 535*), in particular in HIV-infected infants and children (*536*). However, several chronic diseases may mimic respiratory infection, such as asthma, cystic fibrosis, bronchiectasis and immune deficiencies.

The prevalence of childhood asthma ranges from 3% to 20% in different countries, according to the ISAAC report (*33*). Asthma usually starts before the age of 6 years. The most common chronic disease of childhood in many regions of the world, asthma disproportionately burdens many socioeconomically disadvantaged urban communities (*537*).

What GARD will do?

GARD will focus on asthma and rhinitis, the major chronic respiratory diseases in children.

- Asthma is under-diagnosed (*84, 537–539*) and under-treated in children worldwide (*540–542*).
- There are no existing WHO programmes on childhood asthma.
- Diagnosis in young children is difficult, since children at this age cannot cooperate to perform spirometry, and wheezing (a frequent symptom of asthma) can be caused by other diseases.
- Most children with asthma seek medical help during an asthma exacerbation, which primary care physicians often diagnose as respiratory infection.
- Although most cases of childhood asthma can be controlled with medication, many children with asthma still experience persistent symptoms. In low- and middle-income countries, acute

exacerbations of asthma are the leading cause of emergency department visits by paediatric patients.

- Comprehensive guidelines for the diagnosis and treatment of asthma in high-income countries are available (*450, 452*). GARD's asthma education plan should mainly address middle- to low-income countries, as well as low-income areas of high-income countries. Wide experience has already been gained from NAEPP and other programmes on inner city asthma (*60, 65, 75, 408, 543–548*).

Although significant efforts have been made in the past decade to increase awareness of childhood asthma and decrease its burden, there is still an urgent need to develop a simple and realistic asthma education plan to improve skills for identifying and managing asthma in childhood. This plan should be aimed at patients and caregivers, as well as health-care personnel.

In addition to GARD's goals and expected results in relation to adult asthma, specific needs exist in regard to childhood asthma. GARD will support national plans that follow the approach set out below.

Encourage studies on the prevalence of asthma and its risk factors. These studies should cover preschool children, children and adolescents in all countries (including rural areas) and use the respiratory module of the WHO Global Infobase.

Improve the identification of potential asthma patients.

- Many children, particularly in middle-income countries, visit a hospital emergency department for the first time during a severe exacerbation, often because there has been no previous medical diagnosis of asthma.
- In certain countries, physicians diagnose "wheezing" because the term "asthma" is pejorative.
- There is a need to improve the diagnosis and awareness of childhood asthma, particularly in emergency care settings.
- There is a need to improve the diagnosis of asthma, particularly in children under 5 years of age. Asthma often exists in children under 5 years of age, but it is difficult to diagnose and to differentiate from recurrent wheezing (*549*).

Provide a simple guide on how to treat children with asthma in high-low- and middle-income countries. This guide should be distributed in, primary health care centres, emergency rooms and pharmacies.

Educate health-care professionals on how to recognize asthma symptoms, and evaluate and manage a child who might have asthma.

Provide education for patients and caregivers. Educational programmes should be specifically designed for caregivers of infants and young children, school-age children and adolescents.

Prevent smoking initiation during adolescence. Prevention of smoking is a priority goal of any integrated approach to improving lung health, including asthma (*550*).

Box 11 Childhood illnesses

GARD's strategy should always be to aim at integrating actions within primary care. In paediatrics, there are various approaches.

WHO activities in the area of childhood illness

Integrated Management of Childhood Illness (IMCI). **WHO and the United Nations Children's Fund have launched a global initiative to reform the health care received by sick children in low- and middle-income countries in order to prevent deaths (*374, 551–554*). The core intervention of IMCI is the integrated management of the five most important causes of childhood deaths: acute respiratory infections, diarrhoeal diseases, measles, malaria and malnutrition. Like other clinical guidelines, which are increasingly accepted in health systems in low- and middle-income countries, IMCI raises difficult quality issues (*551*).**

Every effort should be made to integrate management of these acute diseases with that of overlapping chronic diseases such as asthma, often exacerbated by acute respiratory infections.

Other activities

National programmes for asthma. **As a part of the Finnish national asthma programme, there is also a national programme on childhood asthma.**

GARD will work on the development of the following tools for the diagnosis and management of childhood asthma:

- A handbook and algorithm on symptoms of asthma in children, to guide professionals in diagnosing asthma without the need for additional tests.
- A simple handbook on how to use laboratory data (where available) to confirm the diagnosis.
- A brochure for day-care providers and schoolteachers.
- A handbook for parents about asthma.
- An educational handbook for children.

24. Identify Policy Implementation Steps

KEY MESSAGES

- **GARD activities need to be implemented at national or regional levels.**
- **National or regional implementation plans needs to be tailored to the health priorities, health-care systems and resources of the country or region.**
- **Implementation plans should involve all stakeholders.**
- **Realistic implementation steps should be proposed.**

GARD supports policy implementation that follows the approach established in *Preventing chronic diseases: a vital investment* (*1*), with three main steps (Figure 21).

- **Implementation step 1** (CORE): interventions that are feasible to implement with existing resources in the short term.
- **Implementation step 2** (EXPANDED): interventions that are possible to implement with a realistically projected increase in, or reallocation of, resources in the medium term.
- **Implementation step 3** (DESIRABLE): evidence-based interventions which are beyond the reach of existing resources.

GARD focuses on the needs of countries, and fosters country-specific initiatives that are tailored to local conditions. In order for GARD's activities to meet the specific needs of countries, national alliances (GARD Country) might be established with a view to providing a coordination role and creating the necessary momentum to face the increasing impact of chronic respiratory diseases (Figure 25). GARD Country could act as an interface between GARD and the ministry of health to create a platform for all parties interested in chronic respiratory diseases in the country. The desired outcome at country level is to initiate or upgrade a programme on the surveillance, prevention and control of chronic respiratory diseases.

Alliances are shaped by the specific health problems and priorities as well as by the economic, political, cultural and social environment in which they work. GARD Country initiator and the core group of interested parties are usually best positioned to decide whether and how to attempt building an alliance at country level, in consultation with the ministry of health and with WHO chronic respiratory diseases and arthritis team that provide secretariat services to GARD.

In order for the national alliance to be sustainable, it should respond to the development needs of the country. GARD Country will respect the country's leadership and support national development and health sector strategies. The following are prerequisites to developing GARD Country:

- The situation of the surveillance, prevention and control of chronic respiratory diseases in the country is analysed.

Figure 25 GARD at country level

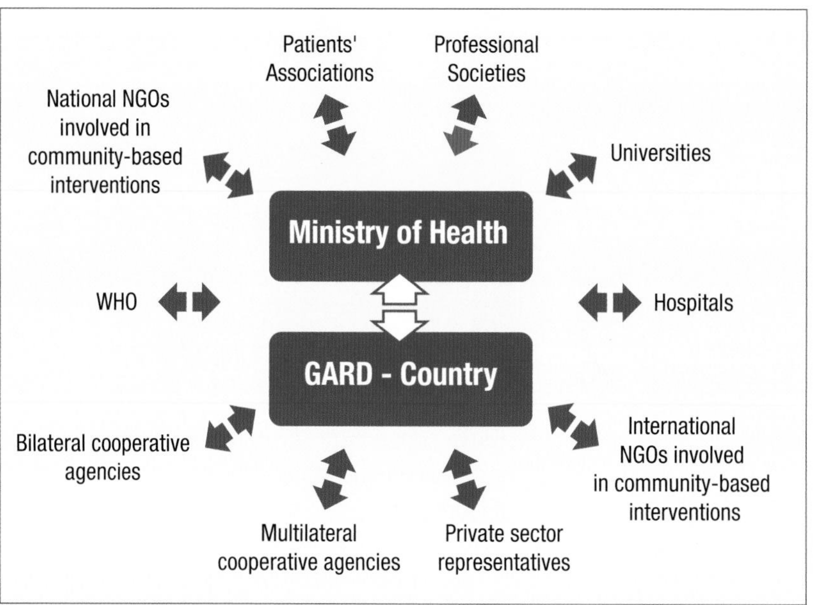

Box 12 Terminology

A GARD country initiator is a person or organization that has developed an initial idea and has taken the first step in formulating the approach of building an alliance at country level. The group of parties that is the most interested in the proposal is the core group of interested parties. Once GARD Country is established, GARD initiator might become GARD Country Coordinator, and the core group of interested parties as well as other interested parties the GARD Country collaborating parties.

- The Ministry of Health of the country is informed about GARD Country and invited to be involved with its development.
- The relevant WHO regional office and the WHO country representative have been informed and invited to be part of GARD Country.

Once the GARD Country initiator has verified that the prerequisites are in place, the following steps are proposed, and can be adapted.

1. Agreeing on a definition of alliance. GARD Country initiator and the core group of interested parties should agree on the term alliance and on its focus.

2. Nominating the GARD Country Coordinator. The WHO chronic respiratory diseases and arthritis team, after consultation with GARD Chairperson, GARD country initiator and the core group of interested parties, might propose GARD Country Coordinator for endorsement by the ministry of health. Alternatively, the ministry of health might nominate GARD country coordinator in agreement with GARD Chairperson and the WHO chronic respiratory diseases and arthritis team.

3. Identifying other potential interested parties. The GARD Country Coordinator, with the help of the core group of interested parties,

should invite as many other interested parties as possible to join GARD Country. After mapping the available resources, GARD Country Coordinator should consider to approach other interested parties, in order to fill the present gaps and help meeting the uncovered needs.

4. Running an exploratory workshop. The GARD Country Coordinator and the focal point within the Ministry of Health should call a workshop including the core group of interested parties and the other potential interested parties. The outcome of this workshop should be an agreement on the goal and objectives, the resources and competencies that each party could bring in, the proposed roles and responsibilities of each party, an outline of the project ideas that could be carried out collaboratively. Once the abovementioned is discussed and agreed upon, a GARD Country Coordinator shall appoint a sub-committee to draft the GARD Country Terms of Reference.

5. Defining the Terms of Reference. The sub-committee should draft the terms of reference of GARD Country. Even if the content of the terms of reference will vary a lot according to the country and the different situations, the draft should include:

    a. general goal: to reduce the burden of chronic respiratory diseases at country level, as part of the global goal to reduce the burden of chronic respiratory diseases worldwide;

    b. technical objectives: these should vary according to the local situation. In general, GARD Country will deal with:

    - coordination of existing activities related to chronic respiratory diseases;
    - exchanging relevant information on chronic respiratory diseases and their risk factors as well as on how to prevent and treat them;
    - advocating on chronic respiratory diseases and their risk factors as well as on how to prevent and treat them;
    - running intervention projects on surveillance, prevention and control of chronic respiratory diseases;
    - generating political commitment at country level;
    - raising additional resources.

The draft of the terms of reference should be circulated to all collaborating parties and to the ministry of health for comments. Once they all agree on the document, they should sign it.

6. Defining the structure: The collaborating parties should find the best way to govern the Alliance according to their various needs.

Here is an example:

a. GARD *Country council* is the plenary body where all GARD collaborating parties are represented. Decisions are taken by consensus. The country coordinator is the Chairperson.

b. GARD *Country planning group* is the proposing body composed of 3 to 5 collaborating parties elected by the council every 2 years. Decisions are taken by consensus. The country coordinator is the Chairperson.

c. GARD *Country secretariat* supports the GARD Country alliance and assists the collaborating parties. It is managed by the GARD Country coordinator and hosted by one of the collaborating parties selected by all the collaborating parties by consensus. The host organization provides a legal umbrella for the alliance which is not a legal entity. The secretariat follows the administrative rules and regulations of the host entity. However, it preserves its own budget and functions

d. GARD Country coordinator should work in close collaboration with GARD focal point within the ministry of health.

7. Reviewing the work of the Alliance: The GARD Country coordinator should review the work of the Alliance on a regular basis. She or he should ask questions on the process, output and outcome. The steps described above are aimed at helping countries to enter in the process of building alliances against chronic respiratory diseases at country level. By adopting this process, GARD Country will be an informed and, therefore, sustainable choice.

REFERENCES

1. Beaglehole R et al. *Preventing chronic diseases: a vital investment.* Geneva, WorldHealth Organization, 2005.

2. Strong K et al. Preventing chronic diseases: how many lives can we save? *The Lancet,*2005, 366:1578–1582.

3. Lee J. Global health improvement and WHO: shaping the future. *The Lancet,* 2003, 366:1821–1824.

4. Srinath RK. Responding to the threat of chronic diseases in India. *The Lancet,* 2005, 366:1744–1749.

5. Wang L. Preventing chronic diseases in China. *The Lancet,* 2005, 366:1821–1824.

6. Murray CJ. Quantifying the burden of disease: the technical basis for disability-adjusted life years. *Bulletin of the World Health Organization,* 1994, 72:429–445.

7. *The World Health Report 2002: reducing risks, promoting healthy life.* Geneva,World Health Organization, 2002.

8. Lyttkens CH. Time to disable DALYs? On the use of disability-adjusted life years in health policy. *European Journal of Health Economics,* 2003, 4:195–202.

9. Beaglehole R, Yach D. Globalization and the prevention and control of non-communicable disease: the neglected chronic diseases of adults. *The Lancet,* 2003, 362:903–908.

10. Prescott E et al. Social position and mortality from respiratory diseases in males and females. *European Respiratory Journal,* 2003, 21:821–826.

11. Epping-Jordan J et al. Preventing chronic diseases: taking stepwise action. *The Lancet,* 2005, 366:1667–1671.

12. Su T, Kouyaté B, Flessa S. Catastrophic household expenditure for health care in a low-income society: a study from Nouna District, Burkina Faso. *Bulletin of the World Health Organization,* 2006, 84:21–27.

13. Bousquet J et al. Management of chronic respiratory and allergic diseases in developing countries. Focus on sub-Saharan Africa. *Allergy,* 2003, 58:265–283.

14. Enarson DA, Ait-Khaled N. Cultural barriers to asthma management. *Pediatric Pulmonology,* 1999, 28:297–300.

15. Masoli M et al. The global burden of asthma: executive summary of the GINA Dissemination Committee Report. *Allergy,* 2004, 59:469–478.

16. Ford ES. The epidemiology of obesity and asthma. *Journal of Allergy and Clinical Immunology,* 2005, 115:897–909.

17. Ait-Khaled N et al. Affordability of inhaled corticosteroids as a potential barrier to treatment of asthma in some developing countries. *The International Journal of Tuberculosis and Lung Disease,* 2000, 4:268–271.

18. Quick JD. Medicines supply in Africa. *British Medical Journal*, 2005, 331:709–710.

19. The Bamako initiative. *The Lancet*, 1988, 2:1177–1178.

20. Kale R. Traditional healers in South Africa: a parallel health care system. *British Medical Journal*, 1995, 310:1182–1185.

21. Siddiqi K, Newell J. Putting evidence into practice in low-resource settings. *Bulletin of the World Health Organization*, 2005, 83:882–883.

22. Fairall LR et al. Effect of educational outreach to nurses on tuberculosis case detection and primary care of respiratory illness: pragmatic cluster randomized controlled trial. *British Medical Journal*, 2005, 331:750–754.

23. Ait-Khaled N, Enarson DA. *Management of asthma. A guide to the essential good of good clinical practice.* 2nd edition. Paris, International Union Against Tuberculosis and Lung Disease, 2005.

24. *WHO strategy for prevention and control of chronic respiratory diseases.* Geneva, World Health Organization, 2002 (http://whqlibdoc.who.int/hq/2002/WHO_MNC_CRA_02.1.pdf, accessed 8 February 2007).

25. *Implementation of the WHO strategy for prevention and control of chronic respiratory diseases: Meeting report 11–12 February 2002, Montpellier.* Geneva, World Health Organization, 2002 (http://whqlibdoc.who.int/HQ/2002/WHO_MNC_CRA_02.2.pdf, accessed 8 February 2007).

26. *Prevention and control of chronic respiratory diseases in low- and middle-income African countries: a preliminary report.* Geneva, World Health Organization, 2003 (http://whqlibdoc.who.int/hq/2003/WHO_NMH_CRA_04.1.pdf, accessed 8 February 2007).

27. *Prevention and control of chronic respiratory diseases at country level: towards a Global Alliance against Chronic Respiratory Diseases.* Geneva, World Health Organization, 2005 (http://whqlibdoc.who.int/hq/2005/WHO_NMH_CHP_CPM_CRA_05.1.pdf, accessed 8 February 2007).

28. Khaltaev N. WHO strategy for prevention and control of chronic obstructive pulmonary disease. *Experimental Lung Research*, 2005, 31:55–56.

29. *International Statistical Classification of Diseases and Related Health Problems,* 10th Revision, Version for 2006. Geneva, World Health Organization, 2006.

30. *World Population Prospects. The 2006 Revision. Highlights.* New York, United Nations, 2007.

31. Ahmad, et al. Age Standardization of Rates: a new WHO standard. *GPE Discussion Paper Series: No.31.* Geneva, World Health Organization, 2007.

32. Halbert R, et al. Global burden of COPD: systematic review and meta-analysis. *European Respiratory Journal*, 2006, 523–532.

33. The International Study of Asthma and Allergies in Childhood (ISAAC) Steering Committee. Worldwide variation in prevalence of symptoms of asthma, allergic rhinoconjunctivitis, and atopic eczema: ISAAC. *The Lancet*, 1998, 351:1225–1232.

34. Janson C et al. The European Community Respiratory Health Survey: what are the main results so far? *European Respiratory Journal*, 2001, 18:598–611.

35. Bauchau V, Durham SR. Epidemiological characterization of the intermittent and persistent types of allergic rhinitis. *Allergy*, 2005, 60:350–353.

36. Bauchau V, Durham SR. Prevalence and rate of diagnosis of allergic rhinitis in Europe. *European Respiratory Journal*, 2004, 24:758–764.

37. Pearce N, Douwes J, Beasley R. Is allergen exposure the major primary cause of asthma? *Thorax*, 2000, 55:424–431.

38. Ross MH, Murray J. Occupational respiratory disease in mining. *Occupational Medicine*, 2004, 54:304–310.

39. Wang XR, Christiani DC. Occupational lung disease in China. *International Journal of Occupational and Environmental Health*, 2003, 9:320–325.

40. Barbosa MM et al. Pulmonary hypertension in schistosomiasis mansoni. *Transactions of the Royal Society of Tropical Medicine and Hygiene*, 1996, 90:663–665.

41. Powars DR et al. Outcome of sickle cell anemia: a 4–decade observational study of 1056 patients. *Medicine*, 2005, 84:363–376.

42. Machado RF, Gladwin MT. Chronic sickle cell lung disease: new insights into the diagnosis, pathogenesis and treatment of pulmonary hypertension. *British Journal of Haematology*, 2005, 129:449–464.

43. Aldashev AA et al. Characterization of high-altitude pulmonary hypertension in the Kyrgyz: association with angiotensin-converting enzyme genotype. *American Journal of Respiratory and Critical Care Medicine*, 2002, 166:1396–1402.

44. Ge RL, Helun G. Current concept of chronic mountain sickness: pulmonary hypertension-related high-altitude heart disease. *Wilderness and Environmental Medicine Journal*, 2001, 12:190–194.

45. Gislason T et al. Prevalence of sleep apnea syndrome among Swedish men–an epidemiological study. *Journal of Clinical Epidemiology*, 1988, 41:571–576.

46. Enright PL et al. Prevalence and correlates of snoring and observed apneas in 5,201 older adults. *Sleep*, 1996, 19:531–538.

47. Ohayon MM et al. Snoring and breathing pauses during sleep: telephone interview survey of a United Kingdom population sample. *British Medical Journal*, 1997, 314:860–863.

48. Larsson LG et al. Gender differences in symptoms related to sleep apnea in a general population and in relation to referral to sleep clinic. *Chest*, 2003, 124:204–211.

49. Ottmani S, et al. *Respiratory care in primary care services. A survey in 9 countries.* Geneva, World Health Organization, 2004.

50. *GINA Report, Global strategy for asthma management and prevention (revised 2006).* Global Initiative for Asthma, 2007.

51. Bousquet J, Khaltaev N, van Cauwenbergue P. Allergic rhinitis and its impact on asthma. *Journal of Allergy and Clinical Immunology*, 2001, 108 (5 Suppl):S147–334.

52. Variations in the prevalence of respiratory symptoms, self-reported asthma attacks, and use of asthma medication in the European Community Respiratory Health Survey (ECRHS). *European Respiratory Journal*, 1996, 9:687–695.

53. Law M et al. Changes in atopy over a quarter of a century, based on cross sectional data at three time periods. *British Medical Journal*, 2005, 330:1187–1188.

54. Rosado-Pinto J, Morais-Almeida M. Asthma in the developing world. *Pediatric Pulmonology*, 2004, 26 (suppl.):66–68.

55. von Hertzen L, Morais-Almeida M. Signs of reversing trends in prevalence of asthma. *Allergy*, 2005, 60:283–292.

56. Linneberg A. Changes in atopy over 25 years: allergy epidemic has spread to old age. *British Medical Journal*, 2005, 331:352.

57. Jarvis D et al. Change in prevalence of IgE sensitization and mean total IgE with age and cohort. *Journal of Allergy and Clinical Immunology*, 2005, 116:675–682.

58. Haahtela T et al. Asthma programme in Finland: a community problem needs community solutions. *Thorax*, 2001, 56:806–814.

59. Ait-Khaled N et al. The Asthma Workshop. Report of a workshop organised by the International Union Against Tuberculosis and Lung Disease, Paris, 15–16 December 2000. *The International Journal of Tuberculosis and Lung Disease*, 2001, 5:973–977.

60. Fischer GB, Camargos PA, Mocelin HT. The burden of asthma in children: a Latin American perspective. *Paediatric Respiratory Reviews*, 2005, 6:8–13.

61. Warman KL, Silver EJ, Stein RE. Asthma symptoms, morbidity, and anti-inflammatory use in inner-city children. *Pediatrics*, 2001, 108:277–282.

62. Bousquet J et al. Quality of life in asthma. Internal consistency and validity of the SF-36 questionnaire. *American Journal of Respiratory and Critical Care Medicine*, 1994, 149:371–375.

63. Leynaert B et al. Quality of life in allergic rhinitis and asthma. A population-based study of young adults. *American Journal of Respiratory and Critical Care Medicine*, 2000, 162:1391–1396.

64. Fighting for breath. A European patient perspective on severe asthma. Brussels, EFA, 2005. (http://www.efanet.org/activities/documents/Fighting_For_Breath1.pdf, accessed 8 February 2007).

65. Tartasky D. Asthma in the inner city: a growing public health problem. *Holistic Nursing Practice*, 1999, 14:37–46.

66. Bonilla S et al. School absenteeism in children with asthma in a Los Angeles inner city school. *Journal of Pediatrics*, 2005, 147:802–806.

67. Guevara JP et al. Effects of educational interventions for self management of asthma in children and adolescents: systematic review and meta-analysis. *British Medical Journal*, 2003, 326:1308–1309.

68. *The world health report 2004: changing history.* Geneva, World Health Organization, 2004.

69. Weiss KB, Sullivan SD. The health economics of asthma and rhinitis. I. Assessing the economic impact. *Journal of Allergy and Clinical Immunology*, 2001, 107:3–8.

70. Sculpher MJ, Price M. Measuring costs and consequences in economic evaluation in asthma. *Respiratory Medicine*, 2003, 97:508–520.

71. Godard P et al. Costs of asthma are correlated with severity: a 1-yr prospective study. *European Respiratory Journal*, 2002, 19:61–67.

72. Yeatts K et al. Health consequences for children with undiagnosed asthma-like symptoms. *Archives of Pediatrics & Adolescent Medicine*, 2003, 157:540–544.

73. Amre DK et al. Socioeconomic status and utilization of health care services among asthmatic children. *Journal of Asthma*, 2002, 39:625–631.

74. Lodha R et al. Social and economic impact of childhood asthma. *Indian Journal of Pediatrics*, 2003, 40:874–879.

75. Evans R et al. A randomized clinical trial to reduce asthma morbidity among inner-city children: results of the National Cooperative Inner-City Asthma Study. *Journal of Pediatrics*, 1999, 135:332–338.

76. Cloutier MM et al. Use of asthma guidelines by primary care providers to reduce hospitalizations and emergency department visits in poor, minority, urban children. *Journal of Pediatrics*, 2005, 146:591–597.

77. Leynaert B et al. Perennial rhinitis: An independent risk factor for asthma in nonatopic subjects: results from the European Community Respiratory Health Survey. *Journal of Allergy and Clinical Immunology*, 1999, 104:301–304.

78. Leynaert B et al. Association between asthma and rhinitis according to atopic sensitization in a population-based study. *Journal of Allergy and Clinical Immunology*, 2004, 113:86–93.

79. Bugiani M et al. Allergic rhinitis and asthma comorbidity in a survey of young adults in Italy. *Allergy*, 2005, 60:165–170.

80. Bousquet et al. Characteristics of intermittent and persistent allergic rhinitis: DREAMS

study group. *Clinical and Experimental Allergy*, 2005, 35:728–732.

81. Strachan D et al. Worldwide variations in prevalence of symptoms of allergic rhinoconjunctivitis in children: the International Study of Asthma and Allergies in Childhood (ISAAC). *Pediatric Allergy and Immunology*, 1997, 8:161–176.

82. Esamai F, Ayaya S, Nyandiko W. Prevalence of asthma, allergic rhinitis and dermatitis in primary school children in Uasin Gishu district, Kenya. *East African Medical Journal*, 2002, 79:514–518.

83. Falade AG et al. Prevalence and severity of symptoms of asthma, allergic rhinoconjunctivitis, and atopic eczema in 6– to 7–year–old Nigerian primary school children: the international study of asthma and allergies in childhood. *Medical Principles and Practice*, 2004, 13:20–25.

84. Hailu S, Tessema T, Silverman M. Prevalence of symptoms of asthma and allergies in schoolchildren in Gondar town and its vicinity, northwest Ethiopia. *Pediatric Pulmonology*, 2003, 35:427–432.

85. Lee SL, Wong W, Lau YL. Increasing prevalence of allergic rhinitis but not asthma among children in Hong Kong from 1995 to 2001 (Phase 3 International Study of Asthma and Allergies in Childhood). *Pediatric Allergy and Immunology*, 2004, 15:72–78.

86. Teeratakulpisarn J, Pairojkul S, Heng S. Survey of the prevalence of asthma, allergic rhinitis and eczema in schoolchildren from Khon Kaen, Northeast Thailand. an ISAAC study. International Study of Asthma and Allergies in Childhood. *Asian Pacific Journal of Allergy and Immunology*, 2000, 18:187–194.

87. Asher MI et al. The burden of symptoms of asthma, allergic rhinoconjunctivitis and atopic eczema in children and adolescents in six New Zealand centres: ISAAC Phase One. *The New Zealand Medical Journal,* 2001, 114:114–120.

88. Akcakaya N et al. Prevalence of bronchial asthma and allergic rhinitis in Istanbul school children. *European Journal of Epidemiology*, 2000, 16:693–699.

89. Vanna AT et al. International Study of Asthma and Allergies in Childhood: validation of the rhinitis symptom questionnaire and prevalence of rhinitis in schoolchildren in Sao Paulo, Brazil. *Pediatric Allergy and Immunology*, 2001, 12:95–101.

90. Shamssain MH, Shamsian N. Prevalence and severity of asthma, rhinitis, and atopic eczema in 13- to 14-year-old schoolchildren from the northeast of England. *Annals of Allergy, Asthma and Immunology*, 2001, 86:428–432.

91. Burney P et al. The distribution of total and specific serum IgE in the European Community Respiratory Health Survey. *Journal of Allergy and Clinical Immunology*, 1997, 99:314–322.

92. Sunyer J et al. Geographic variations in the effect of atopy on asthma in the European Community Respiratory Health Study. *Journal of Allergy and Clinical Immunology*, 2004, 114:1033–1039.

93. Sears MR et al. The relative risks of sensitivity to grass pollen, house dust mite and cat dander in the development of childhood asthma. *Clinical and Experimental Allergy*, 1989, 19:419–424.

94. Wahn U, Von Mutius E. Childhood risk factors for atopy and the importance of early intervention. *Journal of Allergy and Clinical Immunology*, 2001, 107:567–574.

95. Keil T et al. European birth cohort studies on asthma and atopic diseases: I. Comparison study of designs – a GA^{2}LEN initiative. *Allergy*, 2006, 61:221–228.

96. Keil T. European birth cohort studies on asthma and atopic diseases: II. Comparison of outcomes and exposures – a GA^{2}LEN initiative. *Allergy*, 2006, 61:1104–1111.

97. Guerra S et al. Rhinitis as an independent risk factor for adult-onset asthma. *Journal of Allergy and Clinical Immunology*, 2002, 109:419–425.

98. Illi S et al. The natural course of atopic dermatitis from birth to age 7 years and the

association with asthma. *Journal of Allergy and Clinical Immunology*, 2004, 113:925–931.

99. Spergel JM. Atopic march: link to upper airways. *Current Opinion in Allergy and Clinical Immunology*, 2005, 5:17–21.

100. Beeh KM et al. Cigarette smoking, but not sensitization to Alternaria, is associated with severe asthma in urban patients. *Journal of Asthma*, 2001, 38:41–49.

101. Lange P et al. A 15-year follow-up study of ventilatory function in adults with asthma. *New England Journal of Medicine*, 1998, 339:1194–1200.

102. Tomlinson JE et al. Efficacy of low and high dose inhaled corticosteroid in smokers versus non-smokers with mild asthma. *Thorax*, 2005, 60:282–287.

103. Thomson NC, Chaudhuri R, Livingston E. Asthma and cigarette smoking. *European Respiratory Journal*, 2004, 24:822–833.

104. Mathers C, Loncar D. Projections of global mortality and burden of disease from 2002 to 2030. *PLoS Medicine*, 2006, e442.

105. *Global strategy for the diagnosis, management, and prevention of chronic obstructive pulmonary disease. NHLBI/WHO Workshop Report.* National Institutes of Health, National Heart, Lung and Blood Institute, 2001.

106. Celli BR, MacNee W. Standards for the diagnosis and treatment of patients with COPD: a summary of the ATS/ERS position paper. *European Respiratory Journal*, 2004, 23:932–946.

107. *Global strategy for the diagnosis, management, and prevention of chronic obstructive pulmonary disease. NHLBI/WHO Workshop Report. Update 2005.* National Institutes of Health, National Heart, Lung and Blood Institute, 2005.

108. Standards for the diagnosis and care of patients with chronic obstructive pulmonary disease. *American Journal of Respiratory and Critical Care Medicine*, 1995, 152(5 Pt 2): S77–S121.

109. Pauwels R et al. Global strategy for the diagnosis, management, and prevention of chronic obstructive pulmonary disease. NHLBI/WHO Global Initiative for Chronic Obstructive Lung Disease (GOLD) Workshop summary. *American Journal of Respiratory and Critical Care Medicine*, 2001, 163:1256–1276.

110. Guerra S. Overlap of asthma and chronic obstructive pulmonary disease. *Current Opinion in Allergy and Clinical Immunology*, 2005, 11:7–13.

111. *Global strategy for the diagnosis, management, and prevention of chronic obstructive pulmonary disease. NHLBI/WHO Workshop Report. Update 2003.* National Institutes of Health, National Heart, Lung and Blood Institute, 2003.

112. Hogg JC et al. The nature of small-airway obstruction in chronic obstructive pulmonary disease. *New England Journal of Medicine*, 2004, 350:2645–2653.

113. Mannino DM, Doherty DE, Buist SA. Global Initiative on Obstructive Lung Disease (GOLD) classification of lung disease and mortality: findings from the Atherosclerosis Risk in Communities (ARIC) study. *Respiratory Medicine*, 2006, 100:115–122.

114. Chapman K et al. Epidemiology and costs of chronic obstructive pulmonary disease. *European Respiratory Journal*, 2006, 27:188–207.

115. Chan-Yeung M et al. The burden and impact of COPD in Asia and Africa. *The International Journal of Tuberculosis and Lung Disease*, 2004, 8:2–14.

116. Lopez AD, et al. Chronic obstructive pulmonary disease: current burden and future projections. *European Respiratory Journal*, 2006,397–412.

117. Pauwels RA, Rabe KF. Burden and clinical features of chronic obstructive pulmonary disease (COPD). *The Lancet*, 2004, 364:613–620.

118. Lindberg A et al. Prevalence of chronic obstructive pulmonary disease according to

BTS, ERS, GOLD and ATS criteria in relation to doctor's diagnosis, symptoms, age, gender, and smoking habits. *Respiration*, 2005, 72:471–479.

119. Lacasse Y et al. The validity of diagnosing chronic obstructive pulmonary disease from a large administrative database. *Canadian Respiratory Journal*, 2005, 12:251–256.

120. Viegi G et al. Prevalence of airways obstruction in a general population: European Respiratory Society vs American Thoracic Society definition. *Chest*, 2000, 117(5 Supplement 2):339S–345S.

121. Halbert RJ et al. Interpreting COPD prevalence estimates: what is the true burden of disease? *Chest*, 2003, 123:1684–1692.

122. Celli BR et al. Population impact of different definitions of airway obstruction. *European Respiratory Journal*, 2003, 22:268–273.

123. Viegi G et al. The proportional Venn diagram of obstructive lung disease in the Italian general population. *Chest*, 2004, 126:1093–1101.

124. Fukuchi Y et al. COPD in Japan: the Nippon COPD Epidemiology study. *Respirology*, 2004, 9:458–465.

125. Loddenkemper R, Gibson G, Sibille Y. *European lung white book - the first comprehensive survey on respiratory health in Europe.* Huddersfield, European Respiratory Society, 2003.

126. de Marco R et al. An international survey of chronic obstructive pulmonary disease in young adults according to GOLD stages. *Thorax*, 2004, 59:120–125.

127. Mannino DM, Ford ES, Redd SC. Obstructive and restrictive lung disease and functional limitation: data from the Third National Health and Nutrition Examination. *Journal of Internal Medicine*, 2003, 254:540–547.

128. Lange P et al. Chronic obstructive lung disease in Copenhagen: cross-sectional epidemiological aspects. *Journal of Internal Medicine*, 1989, 226:25–32.

129. Dickinson JA et al. Screening older patients for obstructive airways disease in a semi-rural practice. *Thorax*, 1999, 54:501–505.

130. Isoaho R et al. Prevalence of chronic obstructive pulmonary disease in elderly Finns. *Respiratory Medicine*, 1994, 88:571–580.

131. von Hertzen L et al. Airway obstruction in relation to symptoms in chronic respiratory disease – a nationally representative population study. *Respiratory Medicine*, 2000, 94:356–363.

132. Gulsvik A. Prevalence and manifestations of obstructive lung disease in the city of Oslo. *Scandinavian Journal of Respiratory Diseases*, 1979, 60:286–296.

133. Bakke S et al. Prevalence of obstructive lung disease in a general population: relation to occupational title and exposure to some airborne agents. *Thorax*, 1991, 46:863–870.

134. Marco-Jordan L, Martin-Berra J. Chronic obstructive lung disease in the general population. An epidemiologic study performed in Guipuzcoa. *Archivos de Bronconeumología*, 1998, 34:23–27.

135. Pena VS et al. Geographic variations in prevalence and under diagnosis of COPD: results of the IBERPOC multicentre epidemiological study. *Chest*, 2000, 118:981–989.

136. Mueller RE et al. The prevalence of chronic bronchitis, chronic airway obstruction, and respiratory symptoms in a Colorado city. *American Review of Respiratory Diseases*, 1971, 103:209–228.

137. Mannino DM et al. Obstructive lung disease and low lung function in adults in the United States: data from the National Health and Nutrition Examination Survey 1988–1994. *Archives of Internal Medicine*, 2000, 160:1683–1689.

138. Cullen KJ et al. Chronic respiratory disease in a rural community. *The Lancet*, 1968, 2:657–660.

139. Menezes AM, Victora CG, Rigatto M. Prevalence and risk factors for chronic bronchitis in Pelotas, RS, Brazil: a population-based study. *Thorax*, 1994, 49:1217–1221.

140. Menezes AM, Victora CG, Rigatto M. Chronic bronchitis and the type of cigarette smoked. *International Journal of Epidemiology*, 1995, 24:95–99.

141. Littlejohns P, Ebrahim S, Anderson R. Prevalence and diagnosis of chronic respiratory symptoms in adults. *British Medical Journal*, 1989, 298:1556–1560.

142. Magnusson S, Gislason T. Chronic bronchitis in Icelandic males: prevalence, sleep disturbances and quality of life. *Scandinavian Journal of Primary Health Care*, 1999, 17:100–104.

143. Qureshi KA. Domestic smoke pollution and prevalence of chronic bronchitis/asthma in rural area of Kashmir. *Indian Journal of Chest Diseases and Allied Sciences*, 1994, 36:61–72.

144. Pandey RM. Prevalence of chronic bronchitis in a rural community of the Hill Region of Nepal. *Thorax*, 1984, 39:331–336.

145. Cookson JB, Mataka G. Prevalence of chronic bronchitis in Rhodesian Africans. *Thorax*, 1978, 33:328–334.

146. Higgins MW, Keller JB, Metzner HL. Smoking, socioeconomic status, and chronic respiratory disease. *American Review of Respiratory Diseases*, 1977, 116:403–410.

147. Menotti A et al. The relation of chronic diseases to all-cause mortality risk – the Seven Countries Study. *Annals of Internal Medicine*, 1997, 29:135–141.

148. Cerveri I et al. Variations in the prevalence across countries of chronic bronchitis and smoking habits in young adults. *European Respiratory Journal*, 2001, 18:85–92.

149. Chen Y, Breithaupt R, Muhajarine N. Occurence of chronic obstructive pulmonary disease among Canadians and sex-realted risk factors. *Journal of Clinical Epidemiology*, 2000, 53:755–761.

150. Lacasse Y, Brooks D, Goldstein RS. Trends in the epidemiology of COPD in Canada, 1980 to 1995. COPD and Rehabilitation Committee of the Canadian Thoracic Society. *Chest*, 1999, 116:306–313.

151. Meren M et al. Asthma, chronic bronchitis and respiratory symptoms among adults in Estonia according to a postal questionnaire. *Respiratory Medicine*, 2001, 95:954–964.

152. Pallasaho P et al. Increasing prevalence of asthma but not of chronic bronchitis in Finland? Report from the FinEsS-Helsinki Study. *Respiratory Medicine*, 1999, 93:798–809.

153. Lai CK et al. Respiratory symptoms in elderly Chinese living in Hong Kong. *European Respiratory Journal*, 1995, 8:2055–2061.

154. Lundback B et al. Obstructive lung disease in northern Sweden: respiratory symptoms assessed in a postal survey. *European Respiratory Journal*, 1991, 4:257–266.

155. Montnemery P et al. Prevalence of obstructive lung diseases and respiratory symptoms in Southern Sweden. *Respiratory Medicine*, 1998, 92:1337–1345.

156. Lebowitz MD, Knudson RJ, Burrows B. Tucson epidemiologic study of obstructive lung diseases. I: Methodology and prevalence of disease. *American Journal of Epidemiology*, 1975, 102:137–152.

157. Adams P, Hendershot G, Marano M. Current estimates from the National Health Interview Survey, 1996. *Vital Health Statistics*, 1999, 200:1–203.

158. COPD prevalence in 12 Asia-Pacific countries and regions: projections based on the COPD prevalence estimation model. *Respirology*, 2003, 8:192–198.

159. Yang G, et al. Smoking in China: findings of the 1996 National Prevalence Survey. *JAMA: The Journal of the American Medical Association*, 1999, 282:1247–1253.

160. Xu F et al. Prevalence of physician-diagnosed COPD and its association with smoking among urban and rural residents in regional mainland China. *Chest*, 2005, 128:2818–2823.

161. Jindal SK, Aggarwal AN, Gupta D. A review of population studies from India to estimate national burden of chronic obstructive pulmonary disease and its association with smoking. *Indian Journal of Chest Diseases and Allied Sciences*, 2001, 43:139–147.

162. Jindal SK et al. A multicentric study on epidemiology of chronic obstructive pulmonary disease and its relationship with tobacco smoking and environmental tobacco smoke exposure. *Indian Journal of Chest Diseases and Allied Sciences*, 2006, 48:23–29.

163. Jindal SK et al. Tobacco smoking in India: prevalence, quit-rates and respiratory morbidity. *Indian Journal of Chest Diseases and Allied Sciences*, 2006, 48:37–42.

164. Buist SA et al. The Burden of Obstructive Lung Disease initiative (BOLD): Rationale and design. *COPD: Journal of Chronic Obstructive Pulmonary Disease*, 2005, 277–283.

165. Liu SM et al. Epidemiologic analysis of COPD in Guangdong province. *Zhonghua Yi Xue Yi Chuan Xue Za Zhi / Chinese Journal of Medical Genetics*, 2005, 85:747–752.

166. Menezes AM et al. Prevalence of chronic obstructive pulmonary disease and associated factors: the PLATINO Study in Sao Paulo, Brazil. *Cadernos de Saúde Pública*, 2005, 21:1565–1573.

167. Menezes AM, Victora CG, Perez-Padilla R. The Platino project: methodology of a multicenter prevalence survey of chronic obstructive pulmonary disease in major Latin American cities. *BioMed Central Medical Research Methodology*, 2004, 4:15.

168. Menezes AM et al. Chronic obstructive pulmonary disease in five Latin American cities (the PLATINO study): a prevalence study. *The Lancet*, 2005, 366:1875–1881.

169. Soriano JB et al. The proportional Venn diagram of obstructive lung disease: two approximations from the United States and the United Kingdom. *Chest*, 2003, 124:474–481.

170. Zaher C et al. Smoking-related diseases: the importance of COPD. *International Journal of Tuberculosis and Lung Disease*, 2004, 8:1423–1428.

171. Hansell AL, Walk JA, Soriano JB. What do chronic obstructive pulmonary disease patients die from? A multiple cause coding analysis. *European Respiratory Journal*, 2003, 22:809–814.

172. Camilli AE, Robbins DR, Lebowitz MD. Death certificate reporting of confirmed airways obstructive disease. *American Journal of Epidemiology*, 1991, 133:795–800.

173. He J et al. Major causes of death among men and women in China. *New England Journal of Medicine*, 2005, 353:1124–1134.

174. *Morbidity and mortality: 2004 chart book on cardiovascular, lung, and blood diseases.* National Institutes for Health, National Heart, Lung, and Blood Institute; 2004.

175. Jemal A et al. Trends in the leading causes of death in the United States, 1970-2002. *JAMA: The Journal of the American Medical Association*, 2005, 294:1255–1259.

176. *National Heart, Lung, and Blood Institute. Data Fact Sheet: Chronic Obstructive Pulmonary Disease, Vol. 2004.* Department of Health and Human Services, 2004.

177. Sin DD et al. Inhaled corticosteroids and mortality in chronic obstructive pulmonary disease. *Thorax*, 2005, 60:992–997.

178. Murray J, Lopez AD. Mortality by cause for eight regions of the world: Global Burden of Disease Study. *The Lancet*, 1997, 349:1269–1276.

179. Jones P, Lareau S, Mahler DA. Measuring the effects of COPD on the patient. *Respiratory Medicine*, 2005, 99:S11–S18.

180. ZuWallack RL, Haggerty MC, Jones P. Clinically meaningful outcomes in patients with chronic obstructive pulmonary disease. *The American Journal of the Medical Sciences*,

2004, 117: Suppl 12A, 49S–59S.

181. Doll H, Miravitlles M. Health-related QoL in acute exacerbations of chronic bronchitis and chronic obstructive pulmonary disease: a review of the literature. *Pharmacoeconomics*, 2005, 23:345–363.

182. Yeo J, Karimova G, Bansal S. Co-morbidity in older patients with COPD – its impact on health service utilisation and quality of life, a community study. *Age and Ageing*, 2006, 35:33–37.

183. Schmier JK et al. The quality of life impact of acute exacerbations of chronic bronchitis (AECB): a literature review. *Quality of Life Research*, 2005, 14:329–347.

184. Pauwels R et al. COPD exacerbations: the importance of a standard definition. *Respiratory Medicine*, 2006, 98:99–107.

185. MacNee W. Acute exacerbations of COPD. *Swiss Medical Weekly*, 2003, 133 (17-18):247–257.

186. Dolan S, Varkey B. Prognostic factors in chronic obstructive pulmonary disease. *Current Opinion in Pulmonary Medicine*, 2005, 11:149–152.

187. Burney P et al. The pharmacoepidemiology of COPD: recent advances and methodological discussion. *European Respiratory Journal*, 2003, 43:1S–44S.

188. Enfermedad pulmonar obstructiva cronica. Magnitud del problema. Enfermedad pulmonar obstructiva cronica. *Conceptos Generales [General Concepts]*, 1992,57–65.

189. Hilleman DE et al. Pharmacoeconomic evaluation of COPD. *Chest*, 2000, 118:1278–1285.

190. Jacobson L et al. The economic impact of asthma and chronic obstructive pulmonary disease (COPD) in Sweden in 1980 and 1991. *Respiratory Medicine*, 2000, 94:247–255.

191. Wilson L, Devine EB, So K. Direct medical costs of chronic obstructive pulmonary disease: chronic bronchitis and emphysema. *Respiratory Medicine*, 2000, 94:204–213.

192. Rutten-van Molken MP, et al. Current and future medical costs of asthma and chronic obstructive pulmonary disease in The Netherlands. *Respiratory Medicine*, 1999, 93:779–787.

193. Dal-Negro R et al. Global outcomes in Lund Disease Study Group. Cost-of-illness of lung disease in the TriVento Region, Italy: the GOLD study. *Monaldi Archives of Chest Disease*, 2002, 57:3–9.

194. Jansson SA et al. Costs of COPD in Sweden according to disease severity. *Chest*, 2002, 122:1994–2002.

195. Miravitlles M et al. Costs of chronic bronchitis and COPD: a 1-year follow-up study. *Chest*, 2003, 123:784–791.

196. Masa J et al. Costs of chronic obstructive pulmonary disease in Spain: estimation from a population-based study. *Archivos de Bronconeumología*, 2004, 40:72–79.

197. Cotes C. Pharmacoeconomics and the burden of COPD. *Clinical Pulmonary Medicine*, 2005, 12:S19–S21.

198. Mapel DW et al. Predicting the costs of managing patients with chronic obstructive pulmonary disease. *Respiratory Medicine*, 2005, 99:1325–1333.

199. Prescott E, Lange P, Vestbo J. Effect of gender on hospital admissions for asthma and prevalence of self-reported asthma: a prospective study based on a sample of the general population. *Thorax*, 1997, 52:287–289.

200. Hansell AL et al. Validity and interpretation of mortality, health service and survey data on COPD and asthma in England. *European Respiratory Journal*, 2003, 21:279–286.

201. Watson L et al. Predictors of lung function and its decline in mild to moderate COPD in

association with gender: Results from the Euroscop study. *Respiratory Medicine*, 2006, 100:746–753.

202. *WHO Mortality Database*. Geneva, World Health Organization, 2006.

203. Kanner RE et al. Gender difference in airway hyperresponsiveness in smokers with mild COPD. The Lung Health Study. *American Review of Respiratory Diseases*, 1994, 150:956–961.

204. Chen Y, Horne SL, Dosman JA. Increased susceptibility to lung dysfunction in female smokers. *American Review of Respiratory Diseases*, 1991, 143:1224–1230.

205. Chapman K. Chronic obstructive pulmonary disease: are women more susceptible than men? *Clinics in Chest Medicine*, 2004, 25:331–341.

206. Downs SH et al. Accelerated decline in lung function in smoking women with airway obstruction: SAPALDIA 2 cohort study. *Respiratory Research*, 2005, 6:45.

207. Dransfield MT et al. Racial and gender differences in susceptibility to tobacco smoke among patients with chronic obstructive pulmonary disease. *Respiratory Medicine*, 2006, 100:1110-1116.

208. Agusti AG. COPD, a multicomponent disease: implications for management. *Respiratory Medicine*, 2005, 99:670–682.

209. MacNee W. Pulmonary and systemic oxidant/antioxidant imbalance in chronic obstructive pulmonary disease. *Proceedings of the American Thoracic Society*, 2005, 2:50–60.

210. Andreassen H, Vestbo J. Chronic obstructive pulmonary disease as a systemic disease: an epidemiological perspective. *European Respiratory Journal*, 2003, 46 (Suppl): 2–4.

211. Kriegsman DM, Deeg DJ, Stalman WA. Comorbidity of somatic chronic diseases and decline in physical functioning: the Longitudinal Aging Study Amsterdam. *Journal of Clinical Epidemiology*, 2004, 57:55–56.

212. Mikkelsen RL et al. Anxiety and depression in patients with chronic obstructive pulmonary disease (COPD). *Nordic Journal of Psychiatry*, 2004, 58:65–70.

213. Sevenoaks MJ, Stockley RA. Chronic obstructive pulmonary disease, inflammation and co-morbidity – a common inflammatory phenotype? *Respiratory Research*, 2006,70.

214. Sin DD, Man SF. Chronic obstructive pulmonary disease as a risk factor for cardiovascular morbidity and mortality. *Proceedings of the American Thoracic Society*, 2005, 2:8–11.

215. Lyness JM et al. The relationship of medical comorbidity and depression in older, primary care patients. *Psychosomatics*, 2006, 47:435–439.

216. Bolton CE et al. Associated loss of fat-free mass and bone mineral density in chronic obstructive pulmonary disease. *American Journal of Respiratory and Critical Care Medicine*, 2004, 170:1286–1293.

217. Berger JS et al. Comparison of three-year outcomes in blacks versus whites with coronary heart disease following percutaneous coronary intervention. *American Journal of Cardiology*, 2004, 94:647–649.

218. Kjoller E et al. Importance of chronic obstructive pulmonary disease for prognosis and diagnosis of congestive heart failure in patients with acute myocardial infarction. *European Journal of Heart Failure*, 2004, 6:71–77.

219. Sidney S et al. COPD and incident cardiovascular disease hospitalizations and mortality: Kaiser permanente medical care program. *Chest*, 2005, 128:2068–2075.

220. Braunstein JB et al. Noncardiac comorbidity increases preventable hospitalizations and mortality among Medicare beneficiaries with chronic heart failure. *Journal of the American College of Cardiology*, 2003, 42:1226–1233.

221. Petty TL. Are COPD and lung cancer two manifestations of the same disease? *Chest*,

2005, 128:1895–1897.

222. Mannino DM et al. Low lung function and incident lung cancer in the United States: data From the First National Health and Nutrition Examination Survey follow-up. *Archives of Internal Medicine*, 2003, 163:1475–1480.

223. Humphrey LL, Teutsch S, Johnson M. Lung cancer screening with sputum cytologic examination, chest radiography, and computed tomography: an update for the U.S. Preventive Services Task Force. *Annals of Internal Medicine*, 2004, 140:740–753.

224. Deegan PC, McNicholas WT. Pathophysiology of obstructive sleep apnoea. *European Respiratory Journal*, 1995, 8:1161–1178.

225. Young T et al. The occurrence of sleep-disordered breathing among middle-aged adults. *The New England Journal of Medicine*, 1993, 328:1230–1235.

226. Duran J et al. Obstructive sleep apnea-hypopnea and related clinical features in a population-based sample of subjects aged 30 to 70 yr. *American Journal of Respiratory and Critical Care Medicine*, 2001, 163:685–689.

227. Bixler EO et al. Effects of age on sleep apnea in men: I. Prevalence and severity. *American Journal of Respiratory and Critical Care Medicine*, 1998, 157:144–148.

228. Stradling JR, Crosby JH. Predictors and prevalence of obstructive sleep apnoea and snoring in 1001 middle aged men. *Thorax*, 1991, 46:85–90.

229. Bearpark H et al. Snoring and sleep apnea. A population study in Australian men. *American Journal of Respiratory and Critical Care Medicine*, 1995, 151:1459–1465.

230. Ip MS et al. A community study of sleep disorder breathing in middle-aged Chinese men in Hong Kong. *Chest*, 2001, 119:62–69.

231. Ip MS et al. A community study of sleep-disordered breathing in middle-aged Chinese women in Hong Kong: prevalence and gender differences. *Chest*, 2004, 125:127–134.

232. Cistulli PA, Sullivan CE. Sleep apnea in Marfan's syndrome. Increased upper airway collapsibility during sleep. *Chest*, 1995, 108:631–635.

233. Ancoli-Israel S et al. Sleep-disordered breathing in community-dwelling elderly. *Sleep*, 1991, 14:486–495.

234. Cohen-Zion M et al. Changes in cognitive function associated with sleep disordered breathing in older people. *Journal of the American Geriatrics Society*, 2001, 49:1622–1627.

235. Gislason T, Benediktsdottir B. Snoring, apneic episodes, and nocturnal hypoxemia among children 6 months to 6 years old. An epidemiologic study of lower limit of prevalence. *Chest*, 1995, 107:963–966.

236. Marcus CL. Sleep-disordered breathing in children. *American Journal of Respiratory and Critical Care Medicine*, 2001, 164:16–30.

237. Kiely JL, McNicholas WT. Cardiovascular risk factors in patients with obstructive sleep apnoea syndrome. *European Respiratory Journal*, 2000, 16:128–133.

238. Nieto FJ et al. Association of sleep-disordered breathing, sleep apnea, and hypertension in a large community-based study. Sleep Heart Health Study. *JAMA: The Journal of The American Medical Association*, 2000, 283:1829–1836.

239. Peppard PE et al. Prospective study of the association between sleep-disordered breathing and hypertension. *New England Journal of Medicine*, 2000, 342:1378–1384.

240. Shahar E et al. Sleep-disordered breathing and cardiovascular disease: cross-sectional results of the Sleep Heart Health Study. *American Journal of Respiratory and Critical Care Medicine*, 2001, 163:19–25.

241. Peker Y et al. Increased incidence of cardiovascular disease in middle-aged men with obstructive sleep apnea: a 7-year follow-up. *American Journal of Respiratory and Critical Care Medicine*, 2002, 166:159–165.

242. Doherty LS et al. Long-term effects of nasal continuous positive airway pressure therapy on cardiovascular outcomes in sleep apnea syndrome. *Chest*, 2005, 127:2076–2084.

243. Marin JM et al. Long-term cardiovascular outcomes in men with obstructive sleep apnoea-hypopnoea with or without treatment with continuous positive airway pressure: an observational study. *The Lancet*, 2005, 365:1046–1053.

244. Ronald J et al. Healthcare utilization in the 10 years prior to diagnosis in obstructive sleep apnea syndrome patients. *Sleep*, 1999, 22:225–229.

245. Otake K et al. Cardiovascular medication use in patients with undiagnosed obstructive sleep apnea. *Thorax*, 2002, 57:417–422.

246. Bahammam A et al. Healthcare utilization in males with obstructive sleep apnea syndrome two years after diagnosis and treatment. *Sleep*, 1999, 22:740–748.

247. Kapur V et al. The medical cost of undiagnosed sleep apnea. *Sleep*, 1999, 22:749–756.

248. Teran-Santos J, Jimenez-Gomez A, Cordero-Guevara J. The association between sleep apnea and the risk of traffic accidents. *New England Journal of Medicine*, 1999, 340:881–883.

249. Krieger J et al. Public health and medicolegal implications of sleep apnoea. *European Respiratory Journal*, 2002, 20:1594–1609.

250. George CFP. Reduction in motor vehicle collisions following treatment of sleep apnoea with nasal CPAP. *Thorax*, 2001, 56:508–512.

251. Report of a Task Force of the American Academy of Sleep Medicine. Sleep-related breathing disorders in adults: recommendations for syndrome definition and measurement techniques in clinical research. *Sleep*, 1999, 22:667–689.

252. Executive summary on the systematic review and practice parameters for portable monitoring in the investigation of suspected sleep apnea in adults. *American Journal of Respiratory and Critical Care Medicine*, 2004, 169:1160–1163.

253. Cost justification for diagnosis and treatment of obstructive sleep apnea. *Sleep*, 2000, 23:1017–1018.

254. Engleman HM, Douglas NJ. Sleep 4: Sleepiness, cognitive function, and quality of life in obstructive sleep apnoea/hypopnoea syndrome. *Thorax*, 2004, 59:618–622.

255. Naegele B et al. Deficits of cognitive executive functions in patients with sleep apnea syndrome. *Sleep*, 1995, 18:43–52.

256. Arzt M et al. Association of sleep-disordered breathing and the occurrence of stroke. *American Journal of Respiratory and Critical Care Medicine*, 2005, 172:1447–1451.

257. Becker HF et al. Effect of nasal continuous positive airway pressure treatment on blood pressure in patients with obstructive sleep apnea. *Circulation*, 2003, 107:68–73.

258. Simonneau G et al. Clinical classification of pulmonary hypertension. *Journal of the American College of Cardiology*, 2004, 43 (12 Suppl S):5S–12S.

259. Humbert M et al. Risk factors for pulmonary arterial hypertension. *Clinics in Chest Medicine*, 2001, 22:459–475.

260. Naeije R. Pulmonary hypertension and right heart failure in COPD. *Monaldi Archives of Chest Disease*, 2003, 59:250–253.

261. Higenbottam T. Pulmonary hypertension and chronic obstructive pulmonary disease: a case for treatment. *Proceedings of the American Thoracic Society*, 2005, 2:12–19.

262. Maggiorini M, Leon-Velarde F. High-altitude pulmonary hypertension: a pathophysiological entity to different diseases. *European Respiratory Journal*, 2003, 22:1019–1025.

263. Rubin LJ, Badesch DB. Evaluation and management of the patient with pulmonary

arterial hypertension. *Annals of Internal Medicine*, 2005, 143:282–292.

264. Bethlem EP, Schettino G, Carvalho CR. Pulmonary schistosomiasis. *Current Opinion in Pulmonary Medicine*, 1997, 3:361–365.

265. Laosebikan AO, Thomson SR, Naidoo NM. Schistosomal portal hypertension. *Journal of the American College of Surgeons*, 2005, 200:795–806.

266. Lambertucci JR et al. Schistosoma mansoni: assessment of morbidity before and after control. *Acta Tropica*, 2000, 77:101–109.

267. Engels D et al. The global epidemiological situation of schistosomiasis and new approaches to control and research. *Acta Tropica*, 2002, 82:139–146.

268. Gladwin MT et al. Pulmonary hypertension as a risk factor for death in patients with sickle cell disease. *New England Journal of Medicine*, 2004, 350:886–895.

269. Valencia-Flores M et al. Prevalence of pulmonary hypertension and its association with respiratory disturbances in obese patients living at moderately high altitude. *International Journal of Obesity and Related Metabolic Disorders*, 2004, 28:1174–1180.

270. *Fuel for life. Household Energy and Health.* Geneva, World Health Organization, 2006.

271. Bonita R, Howe AL. Older women in an aging world: achieving health across the life course. *World Health Statistics Quarterly*, 1996, 49:134–141.

272. Rehfuess E, Mehta S, Prüss-Ustün A. Assessing Household Solid Fuel Use: Multiple Implications for the Millenium Development Goals. *Environmental Health Perspectives,* 2006, 114:373-378.

273. Warren CW, et al. Global Tobacco Surveillance System (GTSS) collaborative group. Patterns of global tobacco use in young people and implications for future chronic disease burden in adults. *The Lancet*, 2006,749–753.

274. Esson K, Leeder S. *The Millennium Development Goals and Tobacco Control. An opportunity for global partnership.* 2004. Geneva, World Health Organization.

275. Ezzati M, Lopez AD. Estimates of global mortality attributable to smoking in 2000. *The Lancet*, 2003, 362:847–852.

276. *The World Health Report 2003: shaping the future.* Geneva, World Health Organization, 2003.

277. Lopez AD, Collishaw N, Silva V. A descriptive model of the cigarette epidemic in developed countries. *Tobacco Control*, 1994, 3:242–247.

278. Peto R et al. Mortality from smoking worldwide. *British Medical Bulletin*, 1996, 52:12–21.

279. Curbing the epidemic: governments and the economics of tobacco control. 1999. Washington DC, World Bank.

280. Gupta PC et al. Tobacco associated mortality in Mumbai (Bombay) India. Results of the Bombay Cohort Study. *International Journal of Epidemiology*, 2005.

281. *Tobacco: deadly in any form or disguise.* Geneva, World Health Organization, 2006.

282. Gupta PC, Mehta HC. Cohort study of all-cause mortality among tobacco users in Mumbai, India. *Bulletin of the World Health Organization*, 2000, 78:877–883.

283. Neufeld KJ et al. Regular use of alcohol and tobacco in India and its association with age, gender, and poverty. *Drug and Alcohol Dependence*, 2005, 77:283–291.

284. *Report on Carcinogens, Eleventh Edition.* Washington, DC, United States of America Department of Health and Human Services, 2005.

285. Janson C. The effect of passive smoking on respiratory health in children and adults. *International Journal of Tuberculosis and Lung Diseases*, 2004, 8:510–516.

286. Johnson KC. Accumulating evidence on passive and active smoking and breast cancer risk. *International Journal of Cancer*, 2005, 117:619–628.

287. Bonita R et al. Passive smoking as well as active smoking increases the risk of acute stroke. *Tobacco Control*, 1999, 8:156–160.

288. *Proposed Identification of Environmental Tobacco Smoke as a Toxic Air Contaminant, SRP Approved Version, 24 June 2005. Health Effects.* California Environmental Protection Agency (http://www.arb.ca.gov/toxics/ats/finalreport/finalreport.htlm, accesses 4 January 2007).

289. *The Health Consequences of Involuntary Exposure to Tobacco Smoke: A Report of The Surgeon General.* Atlanta, United States of America Department of Health and Human Services, Centers for Diseases Control and Prevention (http://www.cdc.gov/tobacco/sgr/sgr2006/index.htlm, accessed 4 January 2007).

290. Ezzati M et al. Rethinking the "diseases of affluence" paradigm: global patterns of nutritional risks in relation to economic development. *PLoS Medicine*, 2005, 2:e133.

291. Sumer H. et al. The association of biomass fuel combustion on pulmonary function tests in the adult population of Mid-Anatolia. *Sozial- und Präventivmedizin/Social and Preventive Medicine*, 2004, 49:247–253.

292. Viegi G et al. Indoor air pollution and airway disease. *The International Journal of Tuberculosis and Lung Diseases*, 2004, 8:1401–1415.

293. Kunzli N. Biomass fuel makes lungs a decade older – time to take action. *Sozial- und Präventivmedizin/Social and Preventive Medicine*, 2004, 49:233–234.

294. Ekici A et al. Obstructive airway diseases in women exposed to biomass smoke. *Environmental Research*, 2001, 99:93–98.

295. Ezzati M, Kammen D. Indoor air pollution from biomass combustion and acute respiratory infections in Kenya: an exposure–response study. *The Lancet*, 2001, 358:619–624.

296. Mishra V. Indoor air pollution from biomass combustion and acute respiratory illness in preschool age children in Zimbabwe. *International Journal of Epidemiology*, 2003, 32:847–853.

297. Al-Khatib I et al. Impact of housing conditions on the health of the people at al-Ama'ri refugee camp in the West Bank of Palestine. *International Journal of Environmental Health Research*, 2003, 13:315–326.

298. Kiraz K et al. Chronic pulmonary disease in rural women exposed to biomass fumes. *Clinical and Investigative Medicine*, 2003, 26:243–248.

299. Smith KR et al. Indoor air pollution in developing countries and acute lower respiratory infections in children. *Thorax*, 2000, 55:518–532.

300. Shrestha IL, Shrestha SL. Indoor air pollution from biomass fuels and respiratory health of the exposed population in Nepalese households. *International Journal of Occupational and Environmental Health*, 2005, 11:150–160.

301. Golshan M, Faghihi M, Marandi MM. Indoor women jobs and pulmonary risks in rural areas of Isfahan, Iran, 2000. *Respiratory Medicine*, 2002, 6:127.

302. Saha A et al. Pulmonary function and fuel use: a population survey. *Respiratory Research*, 2005, 6:127.

303. Bailis R, Ezzati M, Kammen D. Mortality and greenhouse gas impacts of biomass and petroleum energy futures in Africa. *Science*, 2005, 308:98–103.

304. Orozco-Levi M et al. Wood smoke exposure and risk of chronic obstructive pulmonary disease. *European Respiratory Journal*, 2006, 27:542–546.

305. *Air Quality Guidelines: Global Update 2005.* Geneva, World Health Organization, 2006.

306. What constitutes an adverse health effect of air pollution? Official statement of the

American Thoracic Society. *American Journal of Respiratory and Critical Care Medicine*, 2000, 161:665–673.

307. Hoek G et al. Association between mortality and indicators of traffic-related air pollution in the Netherlands: a cohort study. *The Lancet*, 2002, 360:1203–1209.

308. Pope DW, Dockery DW. Acute health effects of PM10 pollution on symptomatic and asymptomatic children. *American Review of Respiratory Diseases*, 1992, 145:1123–1128.

309. Gauderman WJ et al. The effect of air pollution on lung development from 10 to 18 years of age. *New England Journal of Medicine*, 2004, 351:1057–1067.

310. Yang Q et al. Effect of short-term exposure to low levels of gaseous pollutants on chronic obstructive pulmonary disease hospitalizations. *Environmental Research*, 2005, 99:99–105.

311. Zemp E et al. Long-term ambient air pollution and respiratory symptoms in adults (SAPALDIA study). The SAPALDIA Team. *American Journal of Respiratory and Critical Care Medicine*, 1999, 159:1257–1266.

312. Trasande L, Thurston GD. The role of air pollution in asthma and other pediatric morbidities. *Journal of Allergy and Clinical Immunology*, 2005, 115:689–699.

313. *GINA Report, Global strategy for asthma management and prevention (Revised 2005).* Global Initiative for Asthma, 2005.

314. Tager IB et al. Chronic exposure to ambient ozone and lung function in young adults. *Epidemiology*, 2005, 16:751–759.

315. Cohen AJ et al. The global burden of disease due to outdoor air pollution. *Journal of Toxicology and Environmental Health*, 2005, 68:1301–1307.

316. Cookson W, Moffatt M. Making sense of asthma genes. *New England Journal of Medicine*, 2004, 351:1794–1796.

317. Wong GW et al. Factors associated with difference in prevalence of asthma in children from three cities in China: multicentre epidemiological survey. *British Medical Journal*, 2004, 329:486.

318. Yssel H et al. The role of IgE in asthma. *Clinical and Experimental Allergy*, 1998, 28:104–109.

319. Erwin EA, Platts-Mills TA. Allergens. *Immunology and Allergy Clinics of North America*, 2005, 25:1–14.

320. Sunyer J et al. Geographic variations in the effect of atopy on asthma in the European Community Respiratory Health Study. *Journal of Allergy and Clinical Immunology*, 2004, 114:1033–1039.

321. Camara AA et al. Risk factors for wheezing in a subtropical environment: role of respiratory viruses and allergen sensitization. *Journal of Allergy and Clinical Immunology*, 2004, 113:551–557.

322. Addo-Yobo EO et al. Risk factors for asthma in urban Ghana. *Journal of Allergy and Clinical Immunology*, 2001, 108:363–368.

323. Ndiaye M, Bousquet J. Allergies and parasitoses in sub-Saharan Africa. *Clinical Reviews in Allergy & Immunology*, 2004, 26:105–113.

324. Yazdanbakhsh M, Wahyuni S. The role of helminth infections in protection from atopic disorders. *Current Opinion in Allergy and Clinical Immunology*, 2005, 5:386–391.

325. Rosenstreich DL et al. The role of cockroach allergy and exposure to cockroach allergen in causing morbidity among inner-city children with asthma. *New England Journal of Medicine*, 1997, 336:1356–1363.

326. *Six network meeting of the WHO Collaborating Centres in Occupational Health. Summary report.* 2003. Geneva, World Health Organization.

327. Nelson DI et al. The global burden of selected occupational diseases and injury risks: Methodology and summary. *American Journal of Industrial Medicine*, 2005, 48:400–418.

328. Balmes J et al. American Thoracic Society Statement: occupational contribution to the burden of airway disease. *American Journal of Respiratory and Critical Care Medicine*, 2003, 167:787–797.

329. Gamble JF, Hessel PA, Nicolich M. Relationship between silicosis and lung function. *Scandinavian Journal of Work, Environment & Health*, 2004, 30:5–20.

330. ILO Encyclopedia of Occupational Health and Ss Safety. Geneva, International Labour Organization, 1997.

331. Kazan-Allen L. Asbestos and mesothelioma: worldwide trends. *Lung Cancer*, 2005, 49 Suppl 1:S3–S8.

332. Hessel PA, Gamble JF, McDonald JC. Asbestos, asbestosis, and lung cancer: a critical assessment of the epidemiological evidence. *Thorax*, 2005, 60:433–436.

333. Robinson BW, Musk AW, Lake RA. Malignant mesothelioma. *The Lancet*, 2005, 366:397–408.

334. Davies JC. Silicosis and tuberculosis among South African goldminers –an overview of recent studies and current issues. *South African Medical Journal*, 2001, 91:562–566.

335. Hessel PA, Gamble JF, Nicolich M. Relationship between silicosis and smoking. *Scandinavian Journal of Work, Environment & Health*, 2003, 29:329–336.

336. Vandenplas O, Toren K, Blanc PD. Health and socioeconomic impact of work-related asthma. *European Respiratory Journal*, 2003, 22:689–697.

337. Malo JL et al. Occupational asthma. *Current Opinion in Pulmonary Medicine*, 2004, 10:57–61.

338. Mapp CE et al. Occupational asthma. *American Journal of Respiratory and Critical Care Medicine*, 2005, 172:280–305.

339. Trupin L et al. The occupational burden of chronic obstructive pulmonary disease. *European Respiratory Journal*, 2003, 22:462–469.

340. Driscoll T et al. The global burden of non-malignant respiratory disease due to occupational airborne exposures. *American Journal of Industrial Medicine*, 2005, 48:432–445.

341. Liss GM et al. Hospitalization among workers compensated for occupational asthma. *American Journal of Respiratory and Critical Care Medicine*, 2000, 162:112–118.

342. Loewenson R. Globalization and occupational health: a perspective from southern Africa. *Bulletin of the World Health Organization*, 2001, 79:863–868.

343. Romieu I, Trenga C. Diet and obstructive lung diseases. *Epidemiologic Reviews*, 2001, 23:268–287.

344. *Diet, Nutrition and Prevention of Chronic Diseases. Report of a joint WHO/FAO Expert Consultation.* Geneva, World Health Organization, 2003 (WHO Technical Report Series, No. 916).

345. Ram FS, Ardern KD. Dietary salt reduction or exclusion for allergic asthma. *Cochrane database of systematic reviews*, 2004, 3.

346. McKeever TM, Britton J. Diet and asthma. *American Journal of Respiratory and Critical Care Medicine*, 2004, 170:725–729.

347. Woods R, Thien F, Abramson M. Dietary marine fatty acids (fish oil) for asthma in adults and children. *Cochrane database of systematic reviews*, 2002, 3.

348. Forastiere F et al. Consumption of fresh fruit rich in vitamin C and wheezing symptoms in children. SIDRIA Collaborative Group, Italy (Italian Studies on Respiratory Disorders in

Children and the Environment). *Thorax*, 2000, 55:283–288.

349. Antova T et al. Nutrition and respiratory health in children in six Central and Eastern European countries. *Thorax*, 2003, 58:231–236.

350. Kelly Y, Sacker A, Marmot M. Nutrition and respiratory health in adults: findings from the health survey for Scotland. *European Respiratory Journal*, 2003, 21:664–671.

351. Ram FS, Rowe BH, Kaur B. Vitamin C supplementation for asthma. *Cochrane database of systematic reviews*, 2004, 3.

352. Bergeron C, Boulet LP, Hamid Q. Obesity, allergy and immunology. *Journal of Allergy and Clinical Immunology*, 2005, 115:1102–1104.

353. Hallstrand TS et al. Genetic pleiotropy between asthma and obesity in a community-based sample of twins. *Journal of Allergy and Clinical Immunology*, 2005, 116:1235–1241.

354. Braback L, Hjern A, Rasmussen F. Body mass index, asthma and allergic rhinoconjunctivitis in Swedish conscripts – a national cohort study over three decades. *Respiratory Medicine*, 2005, 99:1010–1014.

355. Mannino DM et al. Boys with high body masses have an increased risk of developing asthma: findings from the National Longitudinal Survey of Youth (NLSY). *International Journal of Obesity*, 2006, 30:6–13.

356. Kim S, Camargo CAJ. Sex-race differences in the relationship between obesity and asthma: the behavioral risk factor surveillance system. *Annals of Epidemiology*, 2003, 13:666–673.

357. Perez-Padilla R et al. Obesity among children residing in Mexico City and its impact on lung function: a comparison with Mexican-Americans. *Archives of Medical Research*, 2006, 37:165–171.

358. Sin DD, Jones RL, Man SF. Obesity is a risk factor for dyspnea but not for airflow obstruction. *Archives of Internal Medicine*, 2002, 162:1477–1481.

359. Lavoie KL et al. Higher BMI is associated with worse asthma control and quality of life but not asthma severity. *Respiratory Medicine*, 2006, 100:648-657.

360. Saint-Pierre P et al. Are overweight asthmatics more difficult to control? *Allergy*, 2006, 61:79–84.

361. Cheng J et al. Calorie controlled diet for chronic asthma. *Cochrane database of systematic reviews*, 2005, 3.

362. *Global Strategy on diet, physical activity and health.* Geneva, World Health Organization, 2004.

363. Prescott E et al. Prognostic value of weight change in chronic obstructive pulmonary disease: results from the Copenhagen City Heart Study. *European Respiratory Journal*, 2002, 20:539–544.

364. Celli BR et al. The body-mass index, airflow obstruction, dyspnea, and exercise capacity index in chronic obstructive pulmonary disease. *New England Journal of Medicine*, 2004, 350:1005–1012.

365. Schols AM. Nutritional and metabolic modulation in chronic obstructive pulmonary disease management. *European Respiratory Journal*, 2003, Suppl November:81s-86s.

366. Calvert J, Burney P. Effect of body mass on exercise-induced bronchospasm and atopy in African children. *Journal of Allergy and Clinical Immunology*, 2005, 116:773–779.

367. Wesley AG. Prolonged after-effects of pneumonia in children. *South African Medical Journal*, 1991, 79:73–76.

368. Sethi GR, Batra V. Bronchiectasis: causes and management. *Indian Journal of Pediatrics*, 2000, 67:133–139.

369. Tiendrebeogo H et al. Cent un cas d'aspergillose pulmonaires en Côte d'Ivoire. *Médecine Tropicale[Tropical Medicine]*, 1982, 42:47–52.

370. Mushegera C, Mbuyi-Muamba JM, Kabemba MJ. Indications and results of pleuropulmonary decortications in the university hospital of Kinshasa. *Acta Chirurgica Belgica*, 1996, 96:217–222.

371. Souilamas R et al. Surgical treatment of active and sequelar forms of pulmonary tuberculosis. *Annals of Thoracic Surgery*, 2001, 71:443–447.

372. Paoletti P et al. Effects of childhood and adolescence-adulthood respiratory infections in a general population. *European Respiratory Journal*, 1989, 2:428–436.

373. Martinez FD. Toward asthma prevention - does all that really matters happen before we learn to read? *New England Journal of Medicine*, 2003, 349:1473–1475.

374. Nelson EA, Olukoya A, Scherpbier RW. Towards an integrated approach to lung health in adolescents in developing countries. *Annals of Tropical Paediatrics*, 2004, 24:117–131.

375. ten Asbroek AH et al. Implementing global knowledge in local practice: a WHO lung health initiative in Nepal. *Health Policy Plan*, 2005, 20:290–301.

376. Veron LJ et al. DOTS expansion: will we reach the 2005 targets? *International Journal of Tuberculosis and Lung Diseases*, 2004, 8:139–146.

377. Armstrong T, Bonita R. Capacity building for an integrated noncommunicable disease risk factor surveillance system in developing countries. *Ethnicity & Disease*, 2003, 13:S13–S18.

378. Burney PG et al. The European Community Respiratory Health Survey. *European Respiratory Journal*, 1994, 7:954–960.

379. Pekkanen J et al. Operational definitions of asthma in studies on its aetiology. *European Respiratory Journal*, 2005, 26:28–35.

380. Pistelli F et al. Usefulness of a compendium of respiratory standard questionnaires for adults (CORSQ). *European Respiratory Review*, 2001, 11:98–102.

381. Pistelli F et al. Appendix 3: Compendium of respiratory standard questionnaires for adults (CORSQ). *European Respiratory Review*, 2001, 11:118–143.

382. Strong KL, Bonita R. Investing in surveillance: a fundamental tool of public health. *Sozialund Präventivmedizin/Social and Preventive Medicine*, 2004, 49:269–275.

383. Piau J-P et al. Questionnaire on health systems and national resources for control of respiratory health in low-income countries. *International Journal of Tuberculosis and Lung Diseases*, 2005, 9:1403–1408.

384. Asher MI et al. International Study of Asthma and Allergies in Childhood (ISAAC): rationale and methods. *European Respiratory Journal*, 1995, 8:483–491.

385. Yach D et al. The global burden of chronic diseases: overcoming impediments to prevention and control. *JAMA: The Journal of the American Medical Association*, 2004, 291:2616–2622.

386. Tang K, Beaglehole R, O'Byrne D. Policy and partnership for health promotion addressing the determinants of health. *Bulletin of the World Health Organization*, 2005, 83:884–885.

387. Kunzli N. The public health relevance of air pollution abatement. *European Respiratory Journal*, 2002, 20:198–209.

388. Rodgers A et al. Distribution of major health risks: findings from the Global Burden of Disease study. *PLoS Medicine*, 2004, 1:e27.

389. Last J. *A Dictionary of Epidemiology.* New York, Oxford University Press, 1995.

390. Borland R et al. Determinants and consequances of smoke-free homes: findings from the International Tobacco Control (ITC) Four Country Survey. *Tobacco Control,* 2006, 15 (suppl 3):71-75.

391. Merom D, Rissel C. Factors associated with smoke free homes in NSW: results from the 1998 NSW health survey. *Australian and New Zealand Journal of Public Health,* 2001, 25:339-345.

392. Borland R et al. Trends in environmental tobacco smoke restrictions in the home in Victoria, Australia. *Tobacco Control,* 1999, 8:226-271.

393. *Protection from exposure to second-hand tobacco smoke. Policy recommendations.* Geneva, World Health Organization, 2007.

394. *Ottawa Charter for Health Promotion.* Geneva, World Health Organization, 1986.

395. Wipfli H et al. Achieving the Framework Convention on Tobacco Control's potential by investing in national capacity. *Tobacco Control*, 2004, 13:433–437.

396. Asher MI et al. World Allergy Organization guidelines for prevention of allergy and allergic asthma. *International Archives of Allergy and Immunology*, 2004, 135:83–92.

397. *Prevention of Allergy and Allergic Asthma.* Geneva, World Health Organization, 2003.

398. Hublet A et al. Smoking in young people with asthma. Journal of Public Health (Oxf) 2007 (Aug 4); Epub ahead of print.

399. Bruce N et al. Impact of improved stoves, house construction and child location on levels of indoor air pollution exposure in young Guatemalan children. *Journal of Exposure Analysis and Environmental Epidemiology*, 2004, 14:S26–S33.

400. Chapman RS et al. Improvement in household stoves and risk of chronic obstructive pulmonary disease in Xuanwei, China: retrospective cohort study. *British Medical Journal*, 2005, 331:1050-1055.

401. El Tayeb Muneer S, Mukhtar Mohamed el W. Adoption of biomass improved cookstoves in a patriarchal society: an example from Sudan. *Science of the Total Environment*, 2003, 307:259–266.

402. Ezzati M, Kammen DM. The health impacts of exposure to indoor air pollution from solid fuels in developing countries: knowledge, gaps, and data needs. *Environmental Health Perspectives*, 2002, 110:1057–1068.

403. Mannan M. Women targeted and women negated. An aspect of the environmental movement in Bangladesh. *Development in practice*, 1996, 6:113–120.

404. Schei M, et al. Childhood asthma and indoor woodsmoke from cooking in Guatemala. *Journal of Exposure Analysis and Environmental Epidemiology*, 2004, 14:S110–S117.

405. Jones CA, Holloway JA, Warner JO. Does atopic disease start in foetal life? *Allergy*, 2000, 55:2–10.

406. Bousquet J et al. Epigenetic inheritance of fetal genes in allergic asthma. *Allergy*, 2004, 59:138–147.

407. Custovic A, Wijk RG. The effectiveness of measures to change the indoor environment in the treatment of allergic rhinitis and asthma: ARIA update (in collaboration with GA^{2}LEN). *Allergy*, 2005, 60:1112–1115.

408. Morgan WJ et al. Results of a home-based environmental intervention among urban children with asthma. *New England Journal of Medicine*, 2004, 351:1068–1080.

409. *American Conference of Governmental and Industrial Hygienists (ACGIH). Threshold Limit Values for Chemical Substances and Physical Agents & Biological Exposure Indices* (http://www.acgih.org, accessed 5 May 2007).

410. Malo JL et al. Natural history of occupational asthma: relevance of type of agent and other factors in the rate of development of symptoms in affected subjects. *Journal of Allergy and Clinical Immunology*, 1992, 90:937–944.

411. Newman Taylor A.J., et al. BOHRF guidelines for occupational asthma. *Thorax*, 2005, 60:364–366.

412. Bernstein I, Storms W. Practice parameters for allergy diagnostic testing. Joint Task Force on Practice Parameters for the Diagnosis and Treatment of Asthma. The American Academy of Allergy, Asthma and Immunology and the American College of Allergy, Asthma and Immunology. *Annals of Allergy, Asthma and Immunology*, 1995, 75:543-625.

413. Li J et al. Algorithm for the diagnosis and management of asthma: a practice parameter update: Joint Task Force on Practice Parameters, representing the American Academy of Allergy, Asthma and Immunology, and the Joint Council of Allergy, Asthma and Immunology. *Annals of Allergy, Asthma and Immunology*, 1998, 81:415–420.

414. Dykewicz M et al. Diagnosis and management of rhinitis: complete guidelines of the Joint Task Force on Practice Parameters in Allergy, Asthma and Immunology. *Annals of Allergy, Asthma and Immunology*, 1998, 81:478–518.

415. Spector S et al. Symptom severity assessment of allergic rhinitis: part 1. *Annals of Allergy, Asthma and Immunology*, 2003, 91:105–114.

416. Brusasco V, Crapo R, Viegi G. Coming together: the ATS/ERS consensus on clinical pulmonary function testing. *European Respiratory Journal*, 2005, 26:1–2.

417. Macintyre N et al. Standardisation of the single-breath determination of carbon monoxide uptake in the lung. *European Respiratory Journal*, 2005, 26:720–735.

418. Miller MR, Dickinson SA, Hickings DJ. The accuracy of portable peak flow meters. *Thorax*, 1992, 47:904–909.

419. Miller MR et al. Standardisation of spirometry. *European Respiratory Journal*, 2005, 26:319–338.

420. Pellegrino R et al. Interpretative strategies for lung function tests. *European Respiratory Journal*, 2005, 26:948–968.

421. Warner JO et al. Standardisation of the measurement of lung volumes. *European Respiratory Journal*, 2005, 26:511–522.

422. Dreborg S et al. Skin tests used in Type I allergy testing. Position Paper of the European Academy of Allergology and Clinical Immunology. *Allergy*, 1988, 44:1–69.

423. Halbert R, Isonaka S. International Primary Care Respiratory Group (IPCRG) Guidelines: Integrating Diagnostic Guidelines for Managing Respiratory Diseases in Primary Care. *Primary Care Respiratory Journal*, 2006, 15:13–19.

424. Levy M et al. International Primary Care Respiratory Group (IPCRG) Guidelines: Diagnosis of Respiratory Diseases in Primary Care. *Primary Care Respiratory Journal*, 2006, 15:i20–i34.

425. Mohangoo AD et al. Prevalence estimates of asthma or COPD from a health interview survey and from general practitioner registration: what's the difference? *European Journal of Public Health*, 2006, 16:101-105.

426. Schneider D, Freeman NC, McGarvey P. Asthma and respiratory dysfunction among urban, primarily Hispanic school children. *Archives of Environmental Health*, 2004, 59:4–13.

427. Wilt TJ et al. Use of Spirometry for Case Finding, Diagnosis, and Management of Chronic Obstructive Pulmonary Disease (COPD). *Evidence report/technology assessment (Summary)*, 2005, 121:1–7.

428. Williams SG et al. Key clinical activities for quality asthma care. Recommendations of the National Asthma Education and Prevention Program. *MMWR Recommendations and Reports*, 2003, 52:1–8.

429. Montnemery P et al. Accuracy of a first diagnosis of asthma in primary health care. *Journal of Family Practice*, 2002, 19:365–368.

430. Rabe KF et al. Worldwide severity and control of asthma in children and adults: The global asthma insights and reality surveys. *Journal of Allergy and Clinical Immunology*, 2004, 114:40–47.

431. O'Dowd LC et al. Attitudes of physicians towards objective measures of airway function in asthma. *American Journal of the Medical Sciences*, 2003, 114:391–396.

432. Yu IT, Wong TW, Li W. Using child reported respiratory symptoms to diagnose asthma in the community. *Archives of Disease in Childhood*, 2004, 89:544–548.

433. Thiadens HA et al. Identifying asthma and chronic obstructive pulmonary disease in patients with persistent cough presenting to general practitioners: descriptive study. *British Medical Journal*, 1998, 316:1286–1290.

434. Soriano JB et al. Validation of general practitioner-diagnosed COPD in the UK General Practice Research Database. *European Journal of Epidemiology*, 2001, 17:1075–1080.

435. Tinkelman DG et al. Symptom-Based Questionnaire for Differentiating COPD and Asthma. *Respiration*, 2006, 73:296-305.

436. Roche N et al. Clinical practice guidelines: medical follow-up of patients with asthma - adults and adolescents. *Respiratory Medicine*, 2005, 99:793–815.

437. Boulet LP et al. Evaluation of asthma control by physicians and patients: comparison with current guidelines. *Canadian Respiratory Journal*, 2002, 9:417–423.

438. Nathan RA et al. Development of the asthma control test: a survey for assessing asthma control. *Journal of Allergy and Clinical Immunology*, 2004, 113:59–65.

439. Juniper EF et al. Measuring asthma control. Clinic questionnaire or daily diary? *American Journal of Respiratory and Critical Care Medicine*, 2000, 162:1330–1334.

440. Juniper EF et al. Identifying 'well-controlled' and 'not well-controlled' asthma using the Asthma Control Questionnaire. *Respiratory Medicine*, 2006, 100:616–621.

441. Gibson PG et al. A research method to induce and examine a mild exacerbation of asthma by withdrawal of inhaled corticosteroid. *Clinical & Experimental Allergy*, 1992, 22:525–532.

442. Freeman D et al. Questions for COPD diagnostic screening in a primary care setting. *Respiratory Medicine*, 2005, 99:1311–1318.

443. Beeh KM et al. Clinical application of a simple questionnaire for the differentiation of asthma and chronic obstructive pulmonary disease. *Respiratory Medicine*, 2004, 98:591–597.

444. Schayck CV et al. Comparison of existing symptom-based questionnaires for identifying COPD in the general practice setting. *Respirology*, 2005, 10:323–333.

445. Price DB et al. COPD Questionnaire Study Group. Scoring system and clinical application of COPD diagnostic questionnaires. *Chest*, 2006, 129:1531-1539.

446. Sprenkle MD et al. The Veterans Short Form 36 questionnaire is predictive of mortality and health-care utilization in a population of veterans with a self-reported diagnosis of asthma or COPD. *Chest*, 2004, 126:81–89.

447. van Schayck CP, Chavannes NH. Detection of asthma and chronic obstructive pulmonary disease in primary care. *European Respiratory Journal*, 2003, 39:16s–22s.

448. *Global initiative for scaling up management of chronic diseases, Report of a WHO Meeting, Cairo, Egypt, 11-13 December 2005.* Geneva, World Health Organization, 2005.

449. *Practical Approach to Lung Health, A primary health care strategy for the integrated management of respiratory conditions in people of five years of age and over.* Geneva, World Health Organization, 2005.

450. Haahtela T, Laitinen LA. Asthma programme in Finland 1994-2004. Report of a Working Group. *Clinical & Experimental Allergy*, 1996, 26 (suppl):1–24.

451. *Programme d'actions, de prévention et de prise en charge de l'asthme. 2002-2005.* (http://www.sante.gouv.fr, accessed 28 Nov 2005).

452. *British guideline on the management of asthma. Thorax*, 2003, 58:i1–i94.

453. Miller MR et al. Severity assessment in asthma: An evolving concept. *Journal of Allergy and Clinical Immunology*, 2005, 116:990–995.

454. *National Asthma Education and Prevention Program (NAEPP), Expert Panel Report 2: Guidelines for the diagnosis and management of asthma- Clinical Practice Guidelines.* Bethesda, United States, National Heart, Lung and Blood Institute, 1997.

455. *National Asthma Education and Prevention Program (NAEPP), Expert Panel Report: Guidelines for the diagnosis and management of asthma- Update on selected topics.* Bethesda, United States, National Heart, Lung and Blood Institute, 2002.

456. Bousquet J, Van Cauwenberge P. ARIA in the pharmacy: management of allergic rhinitis symptoms in the pharmacy. *Allergy*, 2004, 59:373–387.

457. van Schayck CP et al. The IPCRG Guidelines: Developing guidelines for managing chronic respiratory diseases in primary care. *Primary Care Respiratory Journal*, 2006, 15:1–4.

458. O'Byrne P. Asthma Management Guidelines: The Issue of Implementation. *Primary Care Respiratory Journal*, 2006, 15:5–6.

459. Price DB et al. International Primary Care Respiratory Group (IPCRG) guidelines: Management of allergic rhinitis. *Primary Care Respiratory Journal*, 2006, 15:20-34.

460. Bousquet J, Godard P, Grouse L. Global integrated guidelines are needed for respiratory diseases. *Primary Care Respiratory Journal*, 2006, 15:10–12.

461. van-den-Molen T et al. International Primary Care Respiratory Group (IPCRG) Guidelines: Management of Asthma. *Primary Care Respiratory Journal*, 2006, 15:35–47.

462. Higgins BW, Douglas JG. The new BTS/SIGN asthma guidelines: where evidence leads the way. *Thorax*, 2003, 58:98–99.

463. Shivbalan S, Balasubramanian S, Anandnathan K. What do parents of asthmatic children know about asthma?: An Indian perspective. *Indian Journal of Chest Diseases and Allied Sciences*, 2005, 47:81–87.

464. Anderson EW et al. Schools' capacity to help low-income, minority children to manage asthma. *Journal of School Nursing*, 2005, 21:236–242.

465. Henry RL, et al. Randomized controlled trial of a teacher-led asthma education program. *Pediatric pulmonology*, 2004, 38:434–442.

466. Pastore DR, Techow B. Adolescent school-based health care: a description of two sites in their 20th year of service. *Mount Sinai Journal of Medicine*, 2004, 71:191–196.

467. *Global strategy for asthma management and prevention. WHO/NHLBI workshop report.* National Institutes of Health, National Heart, Lung and Blood Institute, 1995.

468. Ressel GW. NAEPP updates guidelines for the diagnosis and management of asthma. *American Family Physician*, 2003, 68:169–170.

469. Lemiere C et al. Adult Asthma Consensus Guidelines Update 2003. *Canadian Respiratory Journal*, 2004, 11:9A–18A.

470. Li J et al. Attaining optimal asthma control: a practice parameter. *Journal of Allergy and Clinical Immunology*, 2005, 116:S3–S11.

471. Bateman ED et al. Can guideline-defined asthma control be achieved? The Gaining Optimal Asthma Control study. *American Journal of Respiratory and Critical Care Medicine*, 2004, 170:836–844.

472. O'Byrne P et al. Budesonide/formoterol combination therapy as both maintenance and reliever medication in asthma. *American Journal of Respiratory and Critical Care Medicine*, 2005, 171:129–136.

473. Sullivan SD et al. Cost-effectiveness analysis of early intervention with budesonide in

mild persistent asthma. *Journal of Allergy and Clinical Immunology*, 2003, 112:1229–1236.

474. Zwar NA et al. General practitioner views on barriers and facilitators to implementation of the Asthma 3+ Visit Plan. *Medical Journal of Australia*, 2005, 183:64–67.

475. Swartz MK, Banasiak NC, Meadows-Oliver M. Barriers to effective pediatric asthma care. *Journal of Pediatric Health Care*, 2005, 19:71–79.

476. Alvarez GG et al. A systematic review of risk factors associated with near-fatal and fatal asthma. *Canadian Respiratory Journal*, 2005, 12:265–270.

477. Gibson G et al. Self-management education and regular practitioner review for adults with asthma. *Cochrane database of systematic reviews*, 2000, 2.

478. Gibson G et al. Limited (information only) patient education programs for adults with asthma. *Cochrane database of systematic reviews*, 2000, 2.

479. Gibson G Powell H. Written action plans for asthma: an evidence-based review of the key components. *Thorax*, 2004, 59:94–99.

480. Toelle BG, Ram FS. Written individualised management plans for asthma in children and adults. *Cochrane database of systematic reviews*, 2004, 2.

481. Yach D. The use and value of qualitative methods in health research in developing countries. *Social Science and Medicine*, 1992, 35:603–612.

482. Laitinen LA, Koskela K. Chronic bronchitis and chronic obstructive pulmonary disease: Finnish National Guidelines for Prevention and Treatment 1998–2007. *Respiratory Medicine*, 1999, 93:297–332.

483. *Programme d'actions, de prévention et de prise en charge de la BPCO, 2001-2005.* (http://www.sante.gouv.fr, accessed 25 November 2005).

484. Fabbri LM, Hurd SS. Global Strategy for the Diagnosis, Management and Prevention of COPD: 2003 update. *European Respiratory Journal*, 2003, 22:1–2.

485. Halpin D. NICE guidance for COPD. *Thorax*, 2006, 59:181–182.

486. National Institute for Clinical Excellence (NICE). Chronic obstructive pulmonary disease: national clinical guideline for management of chronic obstructive pulmonary disease in adults in primary and secondary care. *Thorax*, 2004, 59.

487. MacNee W, Calverley PM. Chronic obstructive pulmonary disease. 7: Management of COPD. *Thorax*, 2003, 58:261–265.

488. Ferguson GT. Recommendations for the management of COPD. *Chest*, 2000, 117:23S–28S.

489. Russi EW et al. Management of chronic obstructive pulmonary disease: the Swiss guidelines. Official Guidelines of the Swiss Respiratory Society. *Swiss Medical Weekly*, 2002, 132:67–78.

490. Bateman ED et al. Guideline for the management of chronic obstructive pulmonary disease (COPD): 2004 revision. *South African Medical Journal*, 2004, 94:559–575.

491. O'Donnell DE et al. State of the Art Compendium: Canadian Thoracic Society recommendations for the management of chronic obstructive pulmonary disease. *Canadian Respiratory Journal*, 2004, 11:7B–59B.

492. Kitamura S. COPD guideline of Japanese Respiratory Society. *Nippon Rinsho*, 2003, 61:2077–2081.

493. Chan-Yeung M t al. Management of chronic obstructive pulmonary disease in Asia and Africa. *International Journal of Tuberculosis and Lung Diseases*, 2004, 8:504–508.

494. Takahashi T et al. Underdiagnosis and undertreatment of COPD in primary care settings. *Respirology*, 2003, 8:504–508.

495. Lindberg A et al. Prevalence and underdiagnosis of COPD by disease severity and the attributable fraction of smoking Report from the Obstructive Lung Disease in Northern Sweden Studies. *Respiratory Medicine*, 2006, 100:264-272.

496. Godtfredsen NS et al. Risk of hospital admission for COPD following smoking cessation and reduction: a Danish population study. *Thorax*, 2002, 57:967–972.

497. Anthonisen NR. The effects of a smoking cessation intervention on 14.5-year mortality: a randomized clinical trial. *Annals of Internal Medicine*, 2005, 142:233–239.

498. Simmons MS et al. Smoking reduction and the rate of decline in FEV(1): results from the Lung Health Study. *European Respiratory Journal*, 2005, 25:1011–1017.

499. Willemse BW et al. Smoking cessation improves both direct and indirect airway hyperresponsiveness in COPD. *European Respiratory Journal*, 2004, 24:391–396.

500. Rennard SI. Treatment of stable chronic obstructive pulmonary disease. *The Lancet*, 2004, 364:791–802.

501. Barnes PJ, Stockley RA. COPD: current therapeutic interventions and future approaches. *European Respiratory Journal*, 2005, 25:1084–1106.

502. Calverley PM. Reducing the frequency and severity of exacerbations of chronic obstructive pulmonary disease. *Proceedings of the American Thoracic Society*, 2004, 1:121–124.

503. Niewoehner DE. Interventions to prevent chronic obstructive pulmonary disease exacerbations. *American Journal of the Medical Sciences*, 2004, 117:41S–48S.

504. Spencer S et al. Impact of preventing exacerbations on deterioration of health status in COPD. *European Respiratory Journal*, 2004, 23:698–702.

505. Poole PJ et al. Influenza vaccine for patients with chronic obstructive pulmonary disease. *Cochrane database of systematic reviews*, 2000, 4.

506. Lacasse Y et al. Pulmonary rehabilitation for chronic obstructive pulmonary disease. *Cochrane database of systematic reviews*, 2002, 3.

507. Puhan MA et al. Respiratory rehabilitation after acute exacerbation of COPD may reduce risk for readmission and mortality – a systematic review. *Respiratory Research*, 2005, 6:54.

508. Cote CG, Celli BR. Pulmonary rehabilitation and the BODE index in COPD. *European Respiratory Journal*, 2005, 26:630–636.

509. Ries AL et al. Effects of pulmonary rehabilitation on physiologic and psychosocial outcomes in patients with chronic obstructive pulmonary disease. *Annals of Internal Medicine*, 1995, 122:823–832.

510. Ries AL. Pulmonary rehabilitation and COPD. *Seminars in Respiratory and Critical Care Medicine*, 2005, 26:133–141.

511. Monninkhof E et al. Economic evaluation of a comprehensive self-management programme in patients with moderate to severe chronic obstructive pulmonary disease. *Chronic Respiratory Disease*, 2004, 1:7–16.

512. Tarpy SP, Celli BR. Long-term oxygen therapy. *New England Journal of Medicine*, 1995, 333:710–714.

513. MacNee W. Prescription of oxygen: still problems after all these years. *American Journal of Respiratory and Critical Care Medicine*, 2005, 172:517–518.

514. Papi A et al. COPD increases the risk of squamous histological subtype in smokers who develop non-small cell lung carcinoma. *Thorax*, 2004, 59:679–681.

515. Mohsenin V. Sleep in chronic obstructive pulmonary disease. *Seminars in Respiratory and Critical Care Medicine*, 2005, 26:109–116.

516. Scanlon PD et al. Loss of bone density with inhaled triamcinolone in Lung Health

Study II. *American Journal of Respiratory and Critical Care Medicine*, 2004, 170:1302–1309.

517. Boot CR et al. Knowledge about asthma and COPD: associations with sick leave, health complaints, functional limitations, adaptation, and perceived control. *Patient Education and Counseling*, 2005, 59:103–109.

518. *Global strategy on occupational health for all: The way to health at work. Recommendation of the second meeting of the WHO Collaborating Centres in Occupational Health.* Beijing, China, World Health Organization, 1995.

519. Gautrin D, Ghezzo H, Malo JL. Rhinoconjunctivitis, bronchial responsiveness, and atopy as determinants for incident non-work-related asthma symptoms in apprentices exposed to high-molecular-weight allergens. *Allergy*, 2003, 58:608–615.

520. Esterhuizen TM et al. Occupational respiratory diseases in South Africa--results from SORDSA, 1997-1999. *South African Medical Journal*, 2001, 91:502–508.

521. Hnizdo E et al. Occupational asthma as identified by the Surveillance of Work-related and Occupational Respiratory Diseases programme in South Africa. *Clinical & Experimental Allergy*, 2001, 31:32–39.

522. Wagner G. *Screening and surveillance of workers exposed to mineral dusts.* Geneva, World Health Organization, 1996.

523. Nicholson PJ et al. Evidence based guidelines for the prevention, identification, and management of occupational asthma. *Journal of Occupational and Environmental Medicine*, 2005, 62:290–299.

524. Ross RM. The clinical diagnosis of asbestosis in this century requires more than a chest radiograph. *Chest*, 2003, 124:1120–1128.

525. Malo JL. Assessment of peak expiratory flow in asthma. *Current Opinion in Pulmonary Medicine*, 1996, 2:75–80.

526. Carroll P, Wachs JE. Managing asthma in the workplace: an overview for occupational health nurses. *American Association of Occupational Health Nurses Journal*, 2004, 52:481–489, quiz 490–491.

527. Humbert M, Sitbon O, Simonneau G. Treatment of arterial pulmonary hypertension. *New England Journal of Medicine*, 2004, 51:1425–1436.

528. Naeije R, Vachiery JL. Medical therapy of pulmonary hypertension. Conventional therapies. *Clinics in Chest Medicine*, 2001, 22:517–527.

529. Sterk PJ et al. The message from the World Asthma Meeting. The Working Groups of the World Asthma Meeting, held in Barcelona, Spain, December 9-13, 1998. *European Respiratory Journal*, 1999, 14:1435–1453.

530. Ait-Khaled N, Enarson D, Bousquet J. Chronic respiratory diseases in developing countries: the burden and strategies for prevention and management. *Bulletin of the World Health Organization*, 2001, 79:971–979.

531. Kunzli N et al. The Global TB Drug Facility: innovative global procurement. *International Journal of Tuberculosis and Lung Diseases*, 2004, 8:130–138.

532. Bilo NE. Do we need an asthma drug facility? *International Journal of Tuberculosis and Lung Diseases*, 2004, 8:391.

533. Coffin SE. Bronchiolitis: in-patient focus. *Pediatric Clinics of North America*, 2005, 52:1047–1057, viii.

534. English M. Impact of bacterial pneumonias on world child health. *Paediatric Respiratory Reviews*, 2000, 1:21–25.

535. Cashat-Cruz M, Morales-Aguirre JJ, Mendoza-Azpiri M. Respiratory tract infections in children in developing countries. *Seminars in Pediatric Infectious Diseases*, 2005, 16:84–92.

536. Graham SM. Non-tuberculosis opportunistic infections and other lung diseases in HIV-infected infants and children. *International Journal of Tuberculosis and Lung Diseases*, 2005, 9:592–602.

537. Gold DR, Wright R. Population disparities in asthma. *Annual Review of Public Health*, 2005, 26:89–113.

538. Okoromah CN, Oviawe O. Is childhood asthma underdiagnosed and undertreated? *Niger Postgraduate Medical Journal*, 2006, 9:221–225.

539. Siersted HC et al. Population based study of risk factors for underdiagnosis of asthma in adolescence: Odense schoolchild study. *British Medical Journal*, 1998, 316:651–655.

540. Bjorkstein B. Unmet needs in the treatment of asthmatic children and adolescents: 2. *Clinical & Experimental Allergy*, 2000, 30:73–76.

541. Ehrlich RI et al. Underrecognition and undertreatment of asthma in Cape Town primary school children. *South African Medical Journal*, 1998, 88:986–994.

542. Riekert KA et al. Caregiver-physician medication concordance and undertreatment of asthma among inner-city children. *Pediatrics*, 2003, 111:e214–e220.

543. Eggleston PA. Environmental causes of asthma in inner city children. The National Cooperative Inner City Asthma Study. *Clinical Reviews in Allergy & Immunology*, 2000, 18:311–324.

544. Federico MJ, Lui AH. Overcoming childhood asthma disparities of the inner-city poor. *Pediatric Clinics of North America*, 2003, 50:655–675, vii.

545. Gellert AR, Gellert SL, Iliffe SR. Prevalence and management of asthma in a London inner city general practice. *British Journal of General Practice*, 1990, 40:197–201.

546. Jones CA et al. A school-based case identification process for identifying inner city children with asthma: the Breathmobile program. *Chest*, 2004, 125:924–934.

547. Velsor-Friedrich B, Pigott T, Srof B. A practitioner-based asthma intervention program with African American inner-city school children. *Journal of Pediatric Health Care*, 2005, 19:163–171.

548. Butz AM et al. Home-based asthma self-management education for inner city children. *Public Health Nursing*, 2005, 22:189–199.

549. Weinberger M. Clinical patterns and natural history of asthma. *Journal of Pediatrics*, 2003, 142:S15-S19, discussion S19–S20.

550. Bundy DG et al. Interpreting subgroup analyses: is a school-based asthma treatment program's effect modified by secondhand smoke exposure? *Archives of Pediatrics & Adolescent Medicine*, 2004, 158:469–471.

551. Heiby JR. Quality improvement and the integrated management of childhood illness: lessons from developed countries. *Joint Commission Journal on Quality Improvement*, 1998, 24:264–279.

552. Moy R. Integrated management of childhood illness (IMCI). *Journal of Tropical Pediatrics*, 1998, 44:190–191.

553. Patwari AK, Raina N. Integrated Management of Childhood Illness (IMCI): a robust strategy. *Indian Journal of Pediatrics*, 2002, 69:41–48.

554. Lulseged S. Integrated management of childhood illness: a review of the Ethiopian experience and prospects for child health. *Ethiopian Medical Journal*, 2002, 40:187–201.

ANNEX

1. Directory of GARD Participants

Name of Organization	Year esta-blished	Journal and Website address	Mission
Allergic Rhinitis and its Impact on Asthma (ARIA).	1999	www.whiar.org	To educate and implement evidence-based management of allergic rhinitis in conjunction with asthma worldwide, through planning, managing, and financing pilot projects to improve the health of broad sectors of the population throughout the world, setting up rural healthcare activities, providing support for preventive diagnostic and therapeutic measures as part of basic healthcare.
ALLERG.O.S	2003		To improve, at a regional level (French Languedoc-Roussillon region), the diagnosis of patients with a suspected severe allergic reactions
American Academy of Allergy, Asthma and Immunology (AAAAI).	1943	*Journal of Allergy & Clinical Immunology* www.aaaai.org	The advancement of the knowledge and practice of allergy, asthma and immunology for optimal patient care.
American College of Allergy, Asthma and Immunology (ACAAI).	1942	*Annals of Allergy, Asthma & Immunology* www.acaai.org	To improve the quality of patient care in allergy and immunology through research, advocacy and professional and public education; maintain and advance diagnostic and therapeutic skills of members; sponsor and conduct educational and scientific programmes and publications; develop and disseminate educational information for members, patients, health-plan purchasers and administrators, and other physicians and health professionals.

Category (Int.Org./NGO/etc.)	Interest sections or assemblies	Number of members/partners and representation by WHO Region
Nongovernmental organization		200: AFRO, AMRO, EMRO, EURO, SEARO, WPRO
Nongovernmental organization, nonprofit organization for clinicians	Missions split into work packages (hymenoptera venom and food anaphylaxis, drug allergy, difficult to control asthma)	70 members (physicians, pharmacists, nurses involved in the network), EURO Region
Nongovernmental organization	7 interest sections: Asthma Diagnosis and Treatment; Basic and Clinical Immunology; Environmental and Occupational Respiratory Diseases; Food Allergy, Dermatologic Diseases and Anaphylaxis; Health Care Education, Delivery and Quality; Mechanisms of Asthma and Allergic Inflammation; Rhinitis, Sinusitis and Ocular Diseases	6000 in Canada, United States of America and 60 other countries: AFRO, AMRO, EMRO, EURO, SEARO, WPRO
Nongovernmental professional association for allergists and immunologists		4900 allergists and immunologists: AMRO and possibly other regions through international affiliate membership

Name of Organization	Year established	Journal and Website address	Mission
American Thoracic Society (ATS).	1905	*American Journal of Respiratory and Critical Care Medicine; American Journal of Respiratory Cell and Molecular Biology; Proceedings of the American Thoracic Society* www.thoracic.org	To prevent and treat respiratory disease through research, education, patient care and advocacy; to decrease morbidity and mortality from respiratory disorders and life-threatening acute illnesses in people of all ages, interacting with national and international organizations that have similar goals.
Asian Allergy and Asthma Foundation (AAAF).	2004	website in preparation	To advance excellent clinical practice of allergic diseases and to reduce their burden through education, training, research, cost effective treatment and public awareness through continuous dialogue with the health ministry and world organizations with the same goals.
Asian Pacific Association of Allergology and Clinical Immunology (APAACI).	1989	www.apaaci.org	To support the development of the discipline of allergy, asthma and clinical immunology in the region; to encourage and assist in forming national societies where none exist; to promote the exchange and progress of knowledge in the region; to study the prevention and treatment of allergy, asthma and immune-mediated diseases specific to the region; to promote exchanges in training programmes between member countries; to help cooperation between clinical and basic research; to develop programmes for public education; to cooperate with other international organizations with similar goals; to disseminate knowledge through international congresses and by other means.
Asian Pacific Society of Respirology (APSR).	1985	*Respirology* www.apsresp.org	To advance and promote knowledge of the respiratory system in health and disease; to strive to encourage research and improve clinical practice through teaching; to increase awareness of health problems in the area and to promote exchange of knowledge among respirologists in the Asia-Pacific region.
Asthma and Allergy Association (AAA).	1991	*Journal Asthme & Allergies Infos* www.asmanet.com	To promote information, medical training and patients' education. Disseminate scientific information; function as a reference body for health organizations and media; encourage and provide training and continuing education. Answer patients'questions through a free hotline.
Danish Lung Health Association (DLHA).	1901	www.lungeforening.dk	To improve prevention and treatment of lung diseases in Denmark and to help patients with these diseases (especially chronic obstructive pulmonary disease) in the country.

Category (Int.Org./NGO/etc.)	Interest sections or assemblies	Number of members/partners and representation by WHO Region
Nongovernmental, nonprofit, international, professional and scientific society for respiratory and critical-care medicine.	12 specialized assemblies	13 000 globally: AFRO, AMRO, EMRO, EURO, SEARO, WPRO
Regional nongovernmental organization		50 members representing all Asian countries: SEARO, WPRO
Association of national societies of allergy and clinical immunology in the Asia-Pacific region		15 national societies in SEARO, WPRO
Regional nongovernmental organization		10,150: SEARO, WPRO
Nongovernmental, nonprofit organization for patients, doctors and health professionnals	sections for asthma, dermatology, paediatrics and allergies to improve information to patients and to promote patients' education.Can propose task forces and joint sessions with other specialist societies.	Over 2 500 members France
National nongovernmental organization		3493 members from the Faroe Islands and Greenland: EURO

Name of Organization	Year esta-blished	Journal and Website address	Mission
Dokkyo University School of Medicine, WHO Collaborating Centre for Prevention and Control of Chronic Respiratory Diseases. (DU-WCC)			Terms of reference as WHO Collaborating Centre; Asia-Pacific Initiative fro Chronic Respiratory Diseases.
European Academy of Allergy and Clinical Immunology (EAACI).	1956	*Allergy (European Journal of Allergy and Clinical Immunology)* www.eaaci.net	To promote basic and clinical research; assess and disseminate scientific information; function as a reference body for other scientific, health and political organizations; encourage and provide training and continuing education; promote good patient care for allergic and immunological diseases.
European Centre for Allergy Research Foundation (ECARF).	2003	www.ecarf.org	To improve knowledge, research and awareness of allergies; decrease the burden of disease in patients and in society through structural research in allergy, spreading of excellence and knowledge among physicians and the public, initiatives for improving patient care, activities for a better quality of life for allergic patients.
European Federation of Allergy and Airways Diseases Patients' Associations (EFA).	1992	www.efanet.org	To improve the quality of life of people with asthma, chronic obstructive pulmonary disease and allergy and of their carers throughout Europe, contributing to a European community that shares the responsibility for substantially reducing the frequency and severity of these conditions and recognizes the social, environmental, economic and health implications.
European Respiratory Society (ERS).	1990	*European Respiratory Journal, European Respiratory Monograph, European Respiratory Review, European Respiratory Topic, ERS Newsletter, Breathe* www.ersnet.org	Promoting research; fostering education; exchanging knowledge; improving patient care.
Finnish Lung Health Association (FILHA).	1907	www.filha.fi	Training and education of management of chronic respiratory diseases; design, implementation of national programmes for diseases (asthma, chronic obstructive pulmonary disease, sleep apnoea), for smoking cessation (since 1994) and implementation of international project (tuberculosis); research, expert networking and human resource development.
Forum of International Respiratory Societies (FIRS).	2002		Advocacy for global respiratory health and identification of new areas for global initiatives. Aims to be attained by the consideration of needs and the proposal of related projects, implemented jointly or individually by the member organizations.

Category (Int.Org./NGO/etc.)	Interest sections or assemblies	Number of members/partners and representation by WHO Region
WHO Collaborating Centre		SEARO, WPRO
Nongovernmental, nonprofit organization for academicians, research investigators and clinicians	Sections for asthma, dermatology, otorhinolaryngology, immunology and paediatrics to improve information exchange and collaboration between scientists within and outside EAACI. Sections can propose task forces and joint sessions with other specialist societies.	39 European national societies, over 3 500 members: EURO
Nongovernmental foundation		Collaboration with Allergy Centre Charité, specialized in clinical work, research and dissemination of knowledge in allergy: EURO
Foundation		Alliance of 41 organizations in 23 countries in Europe representing 250 000 persons: EURO
Nongovernmental, nonprofit international medical organization	10 scientific assemblies serve as forum to present and discuss scientific work at yearly congress	Over 7000 members in 100 countries: AFRO, AMRO, EMRO, EURO, SEARO, WPRO
National nongovernmental organization	WHO collaborating centre	EURO (Finland, Russian Federation, Baltic nations), SEARO (Kyrgyzstan, Mongolia), WPRO (China)
Cooperative union of international professional and scientific societies		Participating organizations include ACCP, ALAT, APSR, ATS, ERS, UNION and ULASTER.

Name of Organization	Year esta-blished	Journal and Website address	Mission
Georgian Respiratory Association (GRA).	2004	*sakartvelos respiraciuli jurnali* (Georgian) www.georanet.org.ge	To promote basic, epidemiological and clinical research in respiratory medicine; to organize regular congresses, conferences, symposia, seminars, scientific meetings, exhibitions and all other clinical and scientific events; to develop and maintain high standards of continuing medical education for medical specialists; to produce scientific publications by the editing, printing, and publishing of reviews, journals, and bulletins to promote, encourage or disseminate research or educational work in the field of respiratory medicine; to produce guidelines on the diagnostic and management of respiratory diseases; to collaborate with other national and international organizations having a similar objectives or similar functions.
Ghent University, WHO Collaborating Centre (GU-WCC) Dept. Respiratory Diseases.	1817	www.ugent.be	To offer high-quality, research-based education; to play an important role in fundamental and applied research; to be an open, pluralistic, international institute with a social responsibility (full mission statement: www.ugent.be/en/ghentuniv/management/mission).
Global Allergy and Asthma European Network (GA2LEN).	2004	www.ga2len.net	To establish an internationally competitive network; to enhance quality and relevance of research and address all aspects of the disease; to decrease the burden of allergy and asthma throughout Europe. Activities consist of integration, coordination of scientific activities and spreading excellence.
Global Initiative for Asthma (GINA).	1991	www.ginasthma.com	Works with health care professionals and public health officials around the world to reduce asthma prevalence, morbidity and mortality. Through evidence-based guidelines for asthma management, and events such as the annual celebration of World Asthma Day, the Global Initiative for Asthma works to improve the lives of people with asthma in every corner of the globe.
Global Initiative for Chronic Obstructive Lung Disease (GOLD).	1998	www.goldcopd.com	Increase awareness of medical community, public health officials and general public that chronic obstructive pulmonary disease is a public health problem; decrease its morbidity and mortality through implementing effective programmes for its diagnosis, management and prevention strategies for use in all countries and promoting studies into the etiology of its increasing prevalence.

Category (Int.Org./NGO/etc.)	Interest sections or assemblies	Number of members/partners and representation by WHO Region
National nongovernmental, nonprofit organization	10 scientific working groups	420 members, 6 branches throughout Georgia; EURO
WHO Collaborating Centre		EURO
Research network in allergy and asthma	Work packages include: nutrition, infection, environment and pollution, occupation, gender sensitization and allergic disease, airway remodelling, clinical care, genetics and genomics	26 leading European teams, EAACI and EFA, one or more centres in each European country: EURO
Programme launched in collaboration with WHO and National Institutes of Health/ National Heart, Lung and Blood Institute	Executive, Science and Dissemination Committees; national launch leaders	AFRO, AMRO, EMRO, EURO, SEARO, WPRO (GARD target countries: Argentina, Brazil, Costa Rica, Portugal, Georgia, Russian Federation, Syrian Arab Republic, Vietnam)
Programme launched in collaboration with WHO and National Institutes of Health/ National Heart, Lung and Blood Institute	Executive, Science and Dissemination Committees. National Launch Leaders	AMRO, EURO

Name of Organization	Year esta-blished	Journal and Website address	Mission
Institute of Neurobiology and Molecular Medicine - Italian National Research Council (INMM-CNR)	1923	www.cnr.it	CNR promotes and carries on research activities, in pursuit of excellence and strategic relevance within the national and international ambit, in the frame of European cooperation and integration. In cooperation with the academic research and with other private and public organizations, CNR ensures the dissemination of results inside the Country, defines, manages and coordinates national and international research programs, in addition to support scientific and research activities of major relevance for the national system. It promotes the valorization, the pre-competitive development and the technological transfer of research results carried on by its own scientific network and by third parties with whom cooperation relationships have been established. It promotes the collaboration in the scientific and technological field, and in the technical regulations field, with organizations and institutions of other Countries, and with supranational organizations in the frame of extra-governmental agreements. It provides, upon request of government authorities, specific skills for the participation of Italy to organizations or international scientific programs of inter-governmental nature. It carries on, through its own program of scholarships and research fellowships, educational and training activities in Ph.D. courses, in advanced after-university specialization courses, and in programs of continuous or recurrent education;
Interdisciplinary Association for Research in Lung Disease (AIMAR).	2001	*Multidisciplinary Respiratory Medicine* www.aimarnetwork.org	To prevent lung disease and promote lung health; to improve the quality of patient care by educating physicians and allied professionals and providing them with programmes and strategies for fighting lung disease such as asthma, chronic obstructive pulmonary disease, infections, tobacco and environmental pollution; to promote research on lung disease; to increase the awareness of public about lung diseases and their risks; to involve all decision-makers in campaigns to reduce environmental and tobacco pollution. To promote and maintain links with all societies and agencies interested in lung health, including patients' organizations, especially in the Mediterranean area.
International Association of Asthmology (INTERASMA).	1954	*Journal of Investigational Allergology & Clinical Immunology, Interasma News newsletter* www.interasma.org	A forum for interdisciplinary discussions among pneumologists, allergists, paediatricians and general practitioners to exchange information on asthma research, practice and management: to focus on all aspects of asthma, bridging the gap between research and clinical practice; to encourage asthma education programmes for all health care professionals, educators and administrators; to improve the quality of life of asthmatics; to decrease the prevalence, morbidity and mortality of asthma.

Category (Int.Org./NGO/etc.)	Interest sections or assemblies	Number of members/partners and representation by WHO Region
Public organization with autonomous rules and regulations, in accordance with the existing laws and the Italian Civil Code	The Institute of Neurobiology and Molecular Medicine (INMM) resulted from the merging of two historical major Institutes of the CNR: The Institute of Neurobiology and The Institute of Molecular Medicine. The Institute is divided in three sections : Neurobiology; Molecular Medicine and Genetics and Molecular Pathophysiology. The research activity of the INMM is mainly focussed on genetic, cellular and molecular mechanisms in health and disease with special reference to allergic and immunologic diseases, diseases of the nervous system, cancerogenesis. The following ongoing/planned studies might be relevant: Allergy and Infections; Innate immunity; IgE sensitisation and inflammation; Tissue remodelling; Biomarkers; Novel drugs; Public Awareness/Education	CNR is made of 108 Institutes with 6962 research workers (2260 Female and 4702 Male).
Nonprofit interdisciplinary association for research in lung disease	Medical areas involved : environmental, general, internal and occupational medicine, intensive care, cardiology, thoracic surgery, radiology, endocrinology, epidemiology, pharmacology, gastroenterology, geriatrics, immunology, infectious diseases, microbiology, neurology, oncology, otolaryngology, paediatrics, pneumology	EURO
International nongovernmental organization	Executive Committee, regional chapters	AMRO, AFRO, EMRO, EURO, WPRO

Name of Organization	Year esta-blished	Journal and Website address	Mission
International Chronic Obstructive Pulmonary Disease Coalition (ICC).	1999	www.internationalcopd.org	To improve care of chronic obstructive pulmonary disease patients through increasing awareness of the disease and an understanding of its diagnosis and management for both carers and patients. To create alliances with professional groups to accomplish these ends. To encourage and support national and regional groups in advocacy efforts toward policy-makers to prioritize chronic obstructive pulmonary disease in research and care.
International Pediatric Respiratory and Allergies Immunological Societies (IPRAIS).	1992		To promote a high standard and clinical service and research for children with respiratory, allergy and immunological disorders. This has been achieved by organising meetings every 2-4 years (Prague 2000, Hong Kong 2003,) and by developing clinical guidelines.
International Primary Care Respiratory Group (IPCRG).	2000	*Primary Care Respiratory Journal* www.theipcrg.org	The primary objects of the charity are to improve public health by raising funds to organise research and reviews into the care, treatment and prevention of respiratory illnesses, diseases and problems in a community setting, and to make available the results of such research for the benefit of the public and healthcare professionals.
International Union Against Tuberculosis and Lung Disease (the UNION).	1956	*International Journal of Tuberculosis & Lung Disease* www.iuatld.org	To prevent and control tuberculosis and lung disease, particularly in low-income countries. To promote national autonomy, within the framework of priorities of each country, by developing, implementing and assessing antituberculosis and respiratory health programmes. To disseminate knowledge on tuberculosis, lung disease, HIV and resulting community health problems in order to alert doctors, decision-makers, opinion-leaders and the general public to the diseases' related dangers. To coordinate, assist and promote the work of its constituent members throughout the world. To establish and maintain close links with WHO, other United Nations organizations, governmental and nongovernmental institutions in health and development sectors.

Category (Int.Org./NGO/etc.)	Interest sections or assemblies	Number of members/partners and representation by WHO Region
Nonprofit corporation; outreach of Global Initiative for Chronic Obstructive Lung Disease and the United States Chronic Obstructive Pulmonary Disease Coalition		220 000 members: AMRO, EMRO, EURO, WPRO
Officially established as a forum, since 1998 IPRAIS became a society		Members from all WHO regions but with particularly strong representation of Asia/Pacific region
Scottish Charity, Company Limited by Guarantee	Sub Committees: Research, Education, Membership, Guidelines and Governance	15 Ordinary Members with voting rights, 19 Associate Members, 2 Internatinal Organisations and 6 Invited specialists
Membership organization with partners in all regions of the world	Scientific groups in asthma, tuberculosis, tobacco prevention, nursing, child lung health	Partners include WHO tuberculosis programme; Stop TB Initiative; Global Fund to Fight AIDS, Tuberculosis and Malaria; Centers for Disease Control and Prevention: AFRO

Name of Organization	Year esta-blished	Journal and Website address	Mission
Italian Society of Respiratory Medicine (SIMER)	1993	*Medicina Toracica* www.simernet.eu	To promote education respiratory medicine and respiratory research, to bridge academic and hospital based respiratory medicine and research by fostering innovation in graduate and post-graduate training, to raise the standards of respiratory care by the production and dissemination of evidence based guidelines and the interaction with the public health political and administrative bodies at the national and regional levels.
Korea Asthma Allergy Foundation (KAF).	2003	www.kaaf.org	To increase the awareness of asthma and allergy to the government and the public and to increase the priority of asthma and allergy in the national health system and to improve the prevention and management of asthma and allergy.
Latin American Thoracic Society (ALAT).	1996	www.alatorax.com	To record and disseminate scientific information about lung diseases; to teach and to promote research on thoracic diseases in Latin America; to stimulate scientific contact between the society's members and other national and international respiratory societies; to develop guidelines for the management of thoracic diseases; to develop scientific departments inside the association; to edit scientific publications.
Libra Project (LIBRA)	2006	*News Letter Progetto Libra* www.progettolibra.it	To raise awareness in public institutions, amongst healthcare workers and the general public on the importance of chronic obstructive diseases which should be considered and dealt with as one of the major problems regarding public health; to make the guidelines known and to change diagnostic and therapeutic standpoints by promoting educational and formative initiatives for healthcare workers; to reduce the number of unrecognized cases and to improve their treatment and optimize costs for the National Health Service whilst improving the quality of diagnostic and therapeutic treatment.
National Centre for Disease Prevention and Control, Ministry of Health, Italy (CCM)	2004	www.ccm.ministerosalute.it	To analyze health risks; coordinate surveillance and active prevention plans of the national alert and response systems; promote and train on the implementation of annual programmes; implement and evaluate annual programmes; network with other national and international health institutions; and information.
National Heart, Lung and Blood Institute (NHLBI), Division of Lung Diseases.		www.nhlbi.nih.gov	Programme on asthma and chronic obstructive pulmonary diseases includes goals on epidemiology, research, genetics and pharmacogenetics, clinical trials, demonstration and education initiatives.

Category (Int.Org./NGO/etc.)	Interest sections or assemblies	Number of members/partners and representation by WHO Region
Scientific, nonprofit organization	Clinical Problems, Respiratory Biology, Intensive and home care, Respiratory Patophysiology, Interventional pneumology, Allergology and Immunology; Infections and Tubercolosis, Epidemiology, Interstitial Lung Disease, Quality in Medicine, Pulmonary Oncology, Sleep Medicine	2100 members EURO Region
National nongovernmental organization	Sections for special task forces such as Burden of Asthma and Computer Assisted Easy Asthma Management and sections for Public Awareness and Education of Physicians and Patients to improve the management of asthma and allergy and to increase priority of asthma and allergy in national health system.	286 members focusing on respiratory medicine and allergy, Republic of Korea
Nongovernmental organization	Asthma, chronic obstructive pulmonary disease, critical pulmonology, endoscopy, interstitial lung diseases, lung infections, thoracic surgery, paediatric pulmonology, pulmonary circulation, respiratory pathophysiology, tuberculosis	5700: AMRO, EURO
Nongovernmental, nonprofit organization for academicians, research investigators and clinicians	LIBRA (Linee Guida Italiane per BPCO, Rinite e Asma – COPD, Rhinitis and Asthma Guidelines) is the joint Italian project for the dissemination of COPD, Rhinitis and Asthma Guidelines which incorporates in one unique structure the Italian GINA, ARIA and GOLD-ERS/ATS projects.	The Executive Committee is made up of the national reporting members of the International Projects: S. Bonini (Rome), G.W. Canonica (Genoa), L.M. Fabbri (Modena), L. Corbetta (Florence), G. Passalacqua (Genoa), P.L. Paggiaro (Pisa). EURO Region
Governmental organization	The Centre is responsible for active prevention of chronic diseases and life styles.	EURO
Governmental organization		Active partner with Global Initiative for Chronic Obstructive Lung Disease and with WHO: AFRO, AMRO, EMRO, EURO, SEARO, WPRO

Name of Organization	Year esta-blished	Journal and Website address	Mission
National Public Health Institute, Finland (KTL).	1911	www.ktl.fi/portal/english	To promote people's possibility of living healthy lives. International collaboration (e.g. multilateral monitoring of trends and determinants in cardiovascular diseases (MONICA) project).
Polish Society of Allergology (PSA).	1982	*International Review of Allergology & Clinical Immunology; Pulmonologia i Alergologia Polska; Alergia Astma Immunologia* www.pta.med.pl	The objective of the society is to organize and support research and scientific works in the filed of experimental and clinical allergology, to associate persons working in these fields and to popularize achievements in pertinent branches of science, as well as to care for a proper level of treatment in allergology.
Portuguese Society of Allergology and Clinical Immunology (SPAIC).	1950	*Revista Portuguesa de Imunoalergologia* www.spaic.pt	To prevent and treat allergic diseases through research, education, patient care and advocacy. To decrease morbidity and mortality from allergic and respiratory disorders, including asthma, in people of all ages, interacting with national and international organizations that have similar goals.
Public Health Agency of Canada (PHAC)	2004	www.phac-aspc.gc.ca	To promote and protect the health of Canadians through leadership, partnership, innovation and action in public health.
Respiratory Society of French Speaking countries (SPLF).	1916	*Revue des maladies respiratoires, Info-Respiration* www.splf.org	To promote all aspects of research in the field of lung diseases; to educate health professionals and patients in order to increase quality of care and awareness; to elaborate programmes for screening, prevention and treatment of lung diseases such as asthma, chronic obstructive pulmonary disease and occupational diseases; to interact with respiratory health officials in order to produce evidence-based guidelines.
Russian Society of Pulmonologists (RSP).		No information available.	
Société Francaise d'Allergologie et d'Immunologie Clinique (SFAIC).	1950	*Revue Française d'Allergologie et d'Immunologie Clinique* www.sfaic.com	To promote basic and clinical research; assess and disseminate scientific information; function as a reference body for other scientific, health and political organizations particularly in French speaking countries; encourage and provide training and continuing education; promote good patient care especially for allergic diseases and also for immunological diseases.

Category (Int.Org./NGO/etc.)	Interest sections or assemblies	Number of members/partners and representation by WHO Region
Governmental institute (under the Ministry of Social Affairs and Health), WHO Collaborating Centre		Finland: EURO
Nonprofit organization	Sections for dermatology, otorhinolaryngology, clinical immunology, eye diseases, young allergologists and paediatrics to improve information exchange and collaboration between scientists within and outside PSA. Sections can propose task forces and joint sessions with other specialist societies	13 Regional Branches, about 1000 members EURO
Nonprofit, nongovernmental, national, professional and scientific society for allergic and respiratory care medicine	12 specialized interest sections: aerobiology, allergy and asthma in sports, asthma, drug allergy, epidemiology, food allergy, immunotherapy, insect venom allergy, latex allergy, primary immunodeficiency, skin allergy, rhinitis	355 active members: EURO
Federal Government	The Centre for Chronic Disease Prevention and Control has several sections including cancer, diabetes, cardiovascular and respiratory disease, and works in the areas of prevention, control, surveillance, risk assessment and policy.	PAHO region
Society	22 working groups involved in the preparation and conduct of a yearly congress	Over 1500 members from various French-speaking countries (central and eastern Europe, African and Asian countries): AFRO, EURO, WPRO
Nongovernmental, nonprofit organization for academicians, research investigators and clinicians	sections for asthma, pulmonology, gastro- enterology, ophtalmology, dermatology, otorhino- laryngology, immunology and paediatrics, occupational diseases to improve information exchange and collaboration between scientists within and outside SFAIC Sections can propose task forces and joint sessions with other specialist societies.	Over 1500 members all over the world but especially EURO Region.

Name of Organization	Year esta-blished	Journal and Website address	Mission
Turkish National Society of Allergy and Clinical Immunology (TNSACI)	1989	*Turkish Journal of Allergy Asthma and Immunology* www.aid.org.tr	Tackle with and try to solve medical, social and economic problems of allergic patients. Conduct investigations into the medical and social aspects of the allergic diseases, and providing support to studies carried out by the government, other associations and organizations in this field. Make propagandas through various publication and broadcasting means and organize conferences in order to elucidate the society in the struggle against allergic diseases and harms caused by them.
Turkish Thoracic Society (TTS).	1992	*Turkish Respiratory Journal* www.toraks.org.tr/english	To provide the most effective scientific methods for prevention, control and treatment of respiratory diseases, and to increase national respiratory health through patient care, research, education and promotion of national policies.
World Allergy Organization (WAO).	1950	*Journal of World Allergy Organization, International Archives of Allergy & Immunology* www.worldallergy.org	To build a global alliance of allergy societies to advance excellence in clinical care, research, education and training.
World Federation of Hydrotherapy and Climatotherapy (FEMTEC).	1937	www.femteconline.com	To explain the medical spa world; to promote it in an international context among States and governing bodies; to encourage international cooperation between spas; to exchange studies, research and practices in the field of hydrotherapy; to promote development of medical spas and climatic resorts among members and worldwide.
World Organization of Family Doctors (WONCA).	1972	www.globalfamilydoctor.com	To improve the quality of life of peoples of the world through defining and promoting its values; by maintaining high standards of care in general practice/family medicine; by promoting personal, comprehensive and continuing care for the individual in the context of the family; by supporting development of academic organizations of general practitioners/family physicians; by providing education to members; by presenting educational, research and service activities of members in other world medical and health organizations.

Category (Int.Org./NGO/etc.)	Interest sections or assemblies	Number of members/partners and representation by WHO Region
Nongovernmental nonprofit organization	Asthma, dermatology, immunotherapy, education, rhinitis, immunology and paediatrics	145 members, EURO Region.
National, nonprofit educational and scientific society	14 scientific working groups	1500 members, 15 branches throughout Turkey: EURO
Worldwide nongovernmental organization; member of Council for International Organizations of Medical Sciences; working relationship with WHO	Federation of 70 national, regional and affiliate organizations	Total individual membership of member societies over 38 000, representing 92 countries: AFRO, AMRO, EMRO, EURO, SEARO, WPRO
Nongovernmental organization in official relations with WHO since 1985	2 500 medical centers involved in activities; once a year, general meeting of Executive Board; meeting of the four permanent committees - medical, economic, technical and social	35 members: thermal and medical spa associations, federations and organizations dealing with spa problems from various countries: AFRO, AMRO, EMRO, EURO, SEARO, WPRO
Nongovernmental organization in official relations with WHO	Governing council meets every three years; regional councils in each region; executive committee meets annually	97 member organizations in 79 countries, total membership over 200 000 general practitioners and family physicians: AFRO, AMRO, EMRO, EURO, SEARO, WPRO